A Paraprof[essional] Handbook

for Working with Students Who Are Visually Impaired

Cyral Miller
Nancy Levack
Editors
Brigitte MaGee
Design

Texas School for the Blind and Visually Impaired

Printed in the United States of America.
First Printing, April 1997

This and the following publications have been sold worldwide and are available from:
Texas School for the Blind and Visually Impaired
Business Office
1100 West 45th Street
Austin, Texas 78756-3494

Independent Living: A Curriculum with Adaptations for Students with Visual Impairments (Vol. I: Social Competence; Vol. II: Self-Care and Maintenance of Personal Environment; Vol. III: Play and Leisure; Supplementary Packet: Assessment and Ongoing Evaluation)
Independent Living: Assessment and Ongoing Evaluation booklet
TAPS: An Orientation and Mobility Curriculum for Students with Visual Impairments (Part I: Curriculum; Part II: Assessment and Ongoing Evaluation booklet)
Low Vision: A Resource Guide with Adaptations for Students with Visual Impairments
Learning Media Assessment of Students with Visual Impairments: A Resource Guide
Teaching Students with Visual and Multiple Impairments: A Resource Guide for Teachers

All the above titles complement this book in educating students with visual impairments and students who have additional disabilities.

Layout, Design, Graphics, and Photographs: Brigitte MaGee, TSBVI Printing:

Library of Congress Cataloging-in-Publication Data
A paraprofessional's handbook for working with students who are visually impaired / Cyral Miller & Nancy Levack, editors.
176 p.
Includes bibliographical references and index.
ISBN 1-880366-21-5
1. Visually handicapped--Education--United States.   2. Visually handicapped--Services for--United States.   3. Teachers of the blind--Training of--United States.   I. Miller, Cyral, 1955-   .   II. Levack, Nancy, 1944-   .
HV1626.P37   1997   97-4158
371.91'1--dc21   CIP

Contents

Daily Living Skills by Nancy Levack & Cyral Miller

Orientation and Mobility Skills by Sharon Trusty & Olga Uriegas

Technology by Debra Leff, Barbara Perdichi, Cecilia Robinson, & Debra Sewell

Adaptation by *Chrissy Cowan*

Students With Multiple Impairments

by Debra Sewell, Millie Smith, Frankie Swift, & Joyce West

Appendix   153

Contributing Writers

Chrissy Cowan, Consultant for the Visually Impaired, Region XIII ESC, Austin

Debra Leff, Consultant for the Visually Impaired, Region XIII ESC, Austin

Nancy Levack, Curriculum Coordinator, TSBVI, Austin

Cyral Miller, Director of Outreach Programs, TSBVI, Austin

Barbara Perdichi, Educational Specialist for the Visually Impaired, Region XII ESC, Waco

Kitty Ramsey, Consultant for the Visually Impaired, Region XIII ESC, Austin

Cecilia Robinson, VI Outreach Education Specialist, TSBVI, Austin

Debra Sewell, VI Outreach Education Specialist, TSBVI, Austin

Millie Smith, VI Outreach Education Specialist, TSBVI, Austin

Frankie Swift, Education Specialist for Visually Impaired, Region XV ESC, San Angelo

Sharon Trusty, Education Specialist for Visually Impaired/ O&M, Region XVII ESC, Lubbock

Olga Uriegas, Visual Impairment, O&M Education Specialist, Region XI ESC, Ft. Worth

Joyce West, Coordinator/Vision Services, Region II ESC, Corpus Christi

Consultants and Reviewers

Craig Axelrod, DB Outreach Education Specialist, TSBVI, Austin

Patty Bearden, Vision Teacher, Northside ISD, San Antonio

Diane Briggs, Vision Teacher, Denton ISD

Peg Brisco, Vision Teacher, TSBVI, Austin

Jim Durkel, DB Outreach Education Specialist, TSBVI, Austin

Jane Erin, Professor, University of Arizona, Department of Special Education

Kathy Geiger, Teacher/Consultant for Visually Impaired, Region V ESC, Beaumont

Martha Gonzales, Paraprofessional, Victoria ISD

Jean Ann Harris, Paraprofessional, Denton ISD

Michelle Kelley Guebel, Specialist for Visually Impaired, Region III ESC, Victoria

Pamala King, Consultant for Students with Visual Impairment, Region VII ESC, Mt. Pleasant

Bevla Lamb, Vision Teacher, Denton ISD

Carol Love, O&M Instructor, UT at Austin

Jeanette Maldonado, Paraprofessional, Northside ISD, San Antonio

Lauren McVeary, O&M Instructor, Region VII ESC, Mt. Pleasant

Sharon Nichols, VI Outreach Education Specialist, TSBVI, Austin

Diane Nousanen, Director/Learning Resource Center, TSBVI, austin

Belinda Oliver, Paraprofessional, Victoria ISD

Nancy Scott, Paraprofessional, Denton ISD

Karen Summers, Vision Teacher, Victoria ISD

Mary Lou Torres, Vision Teacher, Killeen ISD

This list reflects the positions the individuals held when they worked on this publication.

Preface

by Cyral Miller

In 1993, an interest group met to discuss ways to increase the effectiveness of paraprofessionals working with students who are visually impaired. Although it is difficult to document this trend, the general consensus was that the number of assistants in this role has been increasing. The group wanted to try to ensure that the educational assistance being provided by paraprofessionals reflects best practice, both in terms of how their roles are defined and the kinds of support provided to students.

Several paraprofessionals with significant experience in this field identified elements that have helped them be effective, including:

- Vision teachers who are organized

- Well defined roles and responsibilities

- Inclusion of the paraprofessional in team meetings

- Adequate time to prepare material

- Participation in documenting progress on IEP objectives.

In response to a statewide survey, it became apparent that most paraprofessionals had not received formal training on issues relating to vision. Most (56) had received no initial training and nearly half (47) had received no formal training in the past school year. These paraprofessionals were providing direct instruction with consultation from a vision teacher. Primary job duties related to daily living skills, behavior management, recreation and leisure, and facilitating inclusion. Reinforcing skills with assistive devices was also a frequent component of their jobs.

The interest group then looked at existing training material for paraprofessionals. There were numerous references for general training material in special education rules and procedures, but nothing designed specifically for paraprofessionals working with students who are visually impaired.

This handbook grew out of the identified gap between training needs and available material. Hopefully it can be used by vision teachers and paraprofessionals as a way to share basic information needed to work with students who are visually impaired. This information may also be helpful to the wider community of regular teachers, school support staff, parents, and community members. Chapters can be used as needed to support short inservice sessions. Additional reading material for the paraprofessional is listed at the end of each chapter. A more thorough list of printed resources can be found in the Appendix on pages 156-165. While these resource lists are not comprehensive, they reflect selected material specific to visual impairment and relevant to diverse audiences.

Many professionals and paraprofessionals from across Texas contributed to this project as part of the initial interest group and as authors of specific sections. We greatly appreciate the time and effort they contributed to create this handbook.

Students with visual impairments are often fortunate to have paraprofessionals who are well trained as part of the team of educators who support them in successful school careers. We hope this handbook will be of assistance to those team members in making them more comfortable with their unique roles and more knowledgeable about the needs of the students with whom they work.

We want to thank the staff and following students from the Texas School for the Blind and Visually Impaired and the Rosedale Campus of the Austin Independent School District for their cooperation in being photographed to illustrate this book:

Johnny Nolan, Adonia Martinez, Ashly Ford, Keenan Thomas, Randi Beckham, Sara Fennell, Allen Brown, Ricky Lopez, Gabriel Johnson, Chris Sanchez, Courtney Carter, Courtney Jones, Erika Cisneros, Jessica Varnell, Moses Monez, Sara-Anna Treadwell, Mallory Delozier, Ryun Carruthers, Alyssa Rangel, Lindsey Batterbee, Miguel Ruiz, Austin Wells, Duc Tran, Chris Edmerson, John Oxford, Cary Cooper, Juan Vera, David Herrera, Donna Kraft, Casilda, Contreras, and others.

Overview

by
Nancy Levack
Cyral Miller

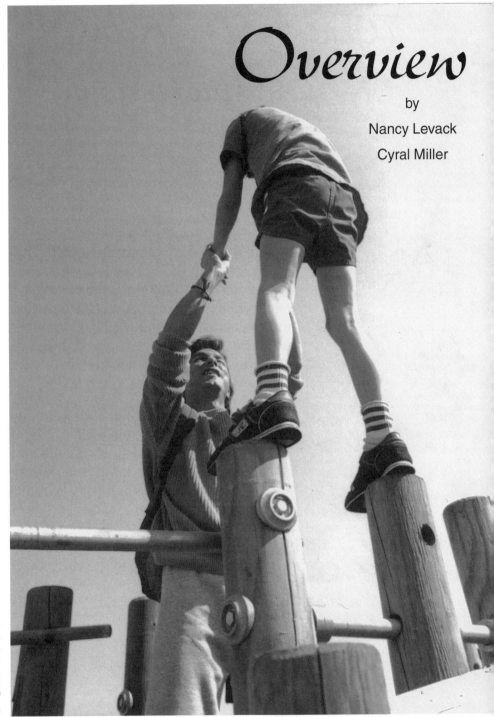

Paraprofessionals have the opportunity to teach in classrooms, on playgrounds, and other on and off campus activities

What Is The Role Of The Paraprofessional?

Definition of Role

Every student in special education has an Individual Education Plan (IEP). This is a legal document which is agreed upon by teachers, administrators and family members at least annually at an Admission, Review, and Dismissal Meeting (ARD). Under the direction of the teachers (VI and classroom), the paraprofessional supports the student in the classroom and implements the goals and objectives of the IEP.

The paraprofessional may be with the student throughout the day and have a broader picture of what is happening in a wide variety of settings. It is important to work closely with the team (e.g., classroom teacher, vision teacher, therapists) to share what is happening with the student.

By virtue of their certification and educational training, the teachers are legally responsible for ensuring that appropriate instruction is provided for the student. The paraprofessional follows those plans while working with the student throughout the day.

A significant challenge to being a paraprofessional in the classroom is providing the appropriate support for students without becoming a barrier between students and their peers. Children can be very adult-oriented and may communicate more with a paraprofessional than with other students. It is the responsibility of a paraprofessional, along with others in the educational team, to look for ways to help students communicate and interact directly with each other.

quote for Paper Eng 125

The paraprofessional frequently helps students getting on and off the schoolbus while reinforcing their orientation and mobility skills.

Roles and Responsibilities of Other Related Service Personnel

Occupational Therapist

- Focuses on fine motor activities, sensory activities and activities of daily living such as eating, dressing, and writing.

- Provides exercises and adaptations for students to increase their independence.

- May work in individual therapy or as a consultant in the classroom.

Physical Therapist

- Focuses on gross motor development.

- Provides exercises and adaptations related to posture and movement.

- Recommends and helps support the use of specialized equipment such as braces, wheelchairs, splints and other adaptive classroom seating.

- May work in individual therapy or as a consultant in the classroom.

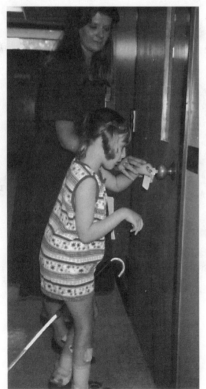

The physical therapist works with the student on motor development using hand-over-hand instruction unlocking a door.

Speech-Language Pathologist

- Focuses on communication skills.

- Provides instruction in and adaptations for articulation, language, voice, fluency, and auditory processing.

- May work in individual therapy or as a consultant in the classroom.

Orientation & Mobility Instructor

- Helps VI children develop skills to move safely and efficiently.

- May recommend ways to modify the home or classroom.

- Teaches the child to use sound, smell, touch, and vision to increase independence.

- May teach the use of a cane or pre-cane device.

- For some students, focuses on the use of distance vision and the use of low vision devices.

- May work individually with a student or groups of students and/or as a consultant in the classroom.

- For some students, gives instruction for independent travel skills in neighborhoods, business areas, malls, and on public transportation.

What Is a Visual Impairment?

Most students who are visually impaired can see some things. In Texas only 448 of the 5,507 students registered as visually impaired in 1996 had no light perception. Some students may see only light and dark shadows, some may see objects best when they are moving, some may see only part of the visual field. An example of a restricted field would be tunnel vision where only the very central part of the visual field is clear. The visual field may be restricted to peripheral vision where some or part of the outside edge of the visual field is clear, such as the sides, top or bottom edges. Some students can see clearly at very limited distances, while others see through an opaque lens and nothing is clear. For some students their vision changes throughout the day depending on fatigue, lighting conditions, and biological factors. It is very important to discuss each student's eye condition with the vision teacher.

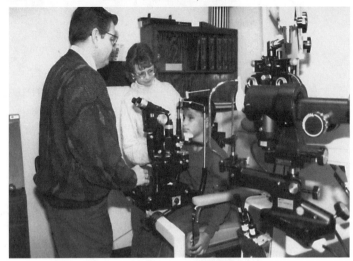

Low vision examinations should be done on a regular basis to determine any changes in vision.

Ask the vision teacher specific questions about:

- The optimum conditions for the student's use of vision.

- The vision teacher's expectations for what kinds of visual tasks the student can do.

Students who have visual impairments with no other disabilities can achieve the same developmental milestones as their sighted peers but there may be some delays in reaching them. It is very important to encourage as much independence as possible for each student. When other disabilities are present, such as cognitive delays, hearing impairments, motor impairments, or emotional disabilities, it is very important to discuss with the vision teacher just how these disabilities affect the student's performance.

The following terms are frequently used when referring to students:

Visual Impairment

In the school setting this identifies a student whose vision is functionally impaired to such a degree that special instructional techniques are needed for optimum learning to take place.

Legally Blind

An acuity of 20/200 or less after correction in the better eye, or a loss in the visual field of 20 degrees or more.

Low Vision

A severe visual impairment after correction. The student does use vision to obtain information with or without optical devices, nonoptical devices and modifications.

Deafblind

A combination of visual and auditory impairments so that special instructional techniques are needed for optimum learning.

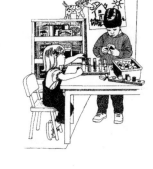

A significant part of programming for students who are visually impaired is ensuring that they are able to efficiently use their senses to obtain information. When students have any vision it is important to teach them when it is most helpful to use their vision, what conditions are most beneficial for seeing, and when necessary, how to interpret what they see.

Touch is an essential sensory mode for students who are visually impaired. Students will need to learn how to locate, explore, manipulate, recognize, compare, and use objects (Smith & Levack, 1996). Another way to look at the sequence of the development of skills in using the sense of touch is:

- Awareness of tactual qualities of objects (e.g., texture, temperature, consistency)

- Recognizing shapes

- Understanding representations (e.g., simple raised line drawings or tactual maps)

- Understanding symbolic tactual systems (e.g., braille) (Griffin & Gerber, 1982).

The sense of hearing also provides essential support for students who are visually impaired. Students may need instruction and programming in attending, localizing and discriminating sound, identifying meaningful environmental sounds, and listening comprehension.

Overview

Language Development

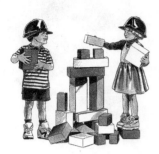

Vision plays an important role in the early stages of development. Vision helps to give meaning to language and provides much information about nonverbal communication. Some children who are visually impaired may be delayed in moving through the stages of language development (Segal, 1993). Four problems that may arise for students who are visually impaired are: verbalisms, echolalia, difficulty with pronouns, and frequent questioning.

Verbalism

Sometimes students who are visually impaired learn to talk about people, objects, and events without having meaningful experiences related to what they are talking about. Also, when students get older and learn to read, they sometimes read about many things and talk about them to others with no real experience or understanding of the object or event. This kind of language is called *verbalism* which is the ability to talk about a subject without the concepts or understanding related to it. It is always important to provide ways for the student to touch and experience the subject and not just hear about it. It is also helpful to ask questions when talking about a subject, to verify that the concepts behind the subject are understood. If they are not understood, problem solve with the teacher how these concepts can be enhanced.

Without careful attention to the development of basic concepts with meaningful langauge students can have a very difficult time understanding increasingly complex material.

Echolalia

When children learn to talk, they spend some time echoing or mimicking phrases or sentences that they do not understand. For some students who are visually impaired, this echolalic phase persists. They may immediately echo what they have just heard or use *delayed echolalia* in which they repeat language heard earlier in association with a particular object or event. There are two important things to consider:

- The speech-language pathologist can evaluate language comprehension if you suspect that the student does not understand the words he is using when communicating.

- If echolalia has been identified, it is helpful to respond to what you suspect the student meant to say, and model appropriate language (e.g., John may use "get your coat" to communicate that he is finished with an activity; the instructor could model "finished" or "John finished" and help him move to a different activity).

If you suspect echolalia, it is important to work closely with the teachers and speech-language pathologist on a plan for how to interpret the student's communications and model appropriate language.

More information about echolalia can be found on page 146.

Using Pronouns

Students who are visually impaired may be delayed in using pronouns correctly. Again, having limited visual feedback makes these words less meaningful. It may be helpful to use names when describing activities rather than using pronouns. For example, "Bobby picks it up," rather than, "I will pick it up."

Frequent Questioning

Some students who are visually impaired ask questions more than usual. Some do this as a way to maintain contact and gain attention because they cannot maintain visual contact with others. It is important to give students other ways of maintaining contact and give feedback if the frequent questioning is a bother to others.

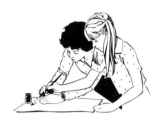

There are times when hand-over-hand assistance is helpful: the instructor guides the student's hands through the activity. However, it is important that students are comfortable with the activity and willing to let you give them guided support. Visually impaired students should not be subjected to having their hands grabbed or placed in or on something without careful preparation and permission. When students are reluctant, allow them to place their hands on the back of yours as you explore or do the task.

There are different levels of prompting and it is always important to use the least amount of prompting needed by the student. In this way you help the student become more independent and able to do tasks without anyone's help. From most (1) to least (6) intensive this hierarchy is:

1. Physical manipulation (e.g., hand-over-hand assistance)

2. Touching but not manipulating some part of the body

3. Giving or showing an object associated with the activity

4. Modeling or gesturing

5. Telling what to do

6. Waiting for the student to perform the action independently. (Smith & Levack, 1996)

Overview

What is Deafblindness?

When students with visual impairments also have auditory impairments, they are identified as deafblind. They can have a range of both visual and hearing abilities. The combined effects of the two sensory losses can significantly change a student's learning needs in several areas. For example, hearing and vision are the distance senses; when both are impaired, gathering information becomes a much more difficult task. The educational team must determine what information the student needs and how to present that in a meaningful way. Communication is a major area of concern. Techniques for relating to others may be different for each deafblind student depending on the circumstances. It is important to discuss each student's communication system(s) with the educational team.

There is a unique role for a paraprofessional working with some students who are deafblind, called an *intervener*. Interveners receive specialized training and will function in ways prescribed by the ARD committee (e.g., to assist the student to actively participate in activities and to provide a supportive and effective communication environment in which the student can learn).

General Suggestions

- Speak directly to the student.

- When you leave students who cannot see, be sure to tell them you are leaving.

- Make corrections in a nonthreatening way with a calm, quiet voice.

- Teach students the importance of facing their conversational partner.

- Let the students know who will be working with them. Describe what they will be doing.

- Make sure that students are not seated near distracting sounds, lights, or noises.

- When leaving students in an unfamiliar setting, guide them to a wall, a chair, or another landmark for orientation.

- For students who are blind, ask for permission to show an object rather than grabbing their hands.

- Do not be afraid to use the words "see" or "look."

- Keeping up with canes can be difficult, especially for young children. Work with the O&M instructor to develop a system for storing and retrieving the cane across all settings.

- Become aware of the lighting and the type of contrast individual students prefer. The O&M instructor or vision teacher will have information on visual functioning. (S. Trusty, 1996)

Additional Reading

Corn, A. L., Cowan, C. M., & Moses, E. (1988). *You seem like a regular kid to me.* New York: American Foundation for the Blind.

First steps: A handbook for teaching young children who are visually impaired. (1993). Los Angeles: Blind Children's Center.

Kekelis, L., & Chernus-Mansfield, N. (1984). *Talk to me: A language guide for parents of blind children.* Los Angeles: Blind Children's Center.

Kekelis, L., Chernus-Mansfield, N., & Hayashi, D. (1985). *Talk to me II: Common concerns.* Los Angeles: Blind Children's Center.

Torres, I., & Corn, A. L. (1990). *When you have a visually impaired child in your classroom: Suggestions for teachers.* 2nd ed. New York: American Foundation for the Blind.

References

Griffin, H. C., & Gerber, P. J. (1982). Tactual development and its implications for the education of blind children. *Education of the Visually Handicapped, 13,* 4, 116-123.

Hatfield, E. M. (1975). Why are they blind? *The Sight-Saving Review, 45,* 1, 3-22.

Segal, J. (1993). Chapter 6, Speech and language development. In *First steps: A handbook for teaching young children who are visually impaired.* Los Angeles: Blind Children's Center.

Smith, M., & Levack, N. (1996). *Teaching students with visual and multiple impairments: A resource guide.* Austin: Texas School for the Blind and Visually Impaired.

Trusty, S. (1996). Personal correspondence.

Overview

Social Skills

by Kitty Ramsey

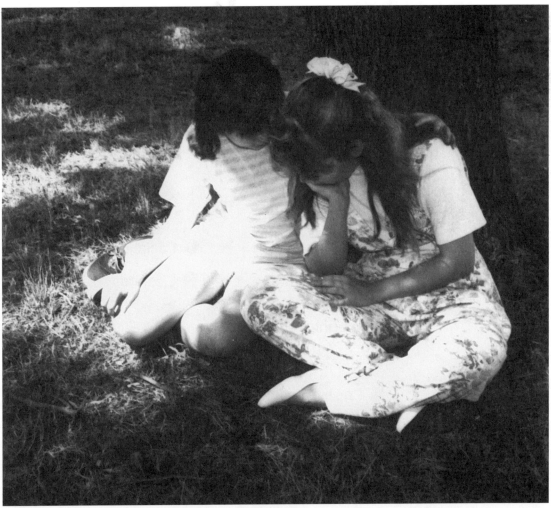

Friendships are important to all children. Paraprofessionals can help students establish friendships.

What Are Social Skills?

Social skills are learned behaviors which enable us to have positive, successful interactions with our family, friends, community, and coworkers.

The following categories address some of the social skills activities that might be taught within a school program:

Body Language

● Eye contact   ● Facial expressions

● Body posture   ● Gestures

Communication Skills

● Initiating interactions   ● Conversation skills

● Positive communication with others

Cooperative Skills

● Joining and participating in group activities successfully

Why Are They Important?

Social skills are important because they:

- Help us develop a sense of independence, responsibility, and cooperation.

- Contribute to the development of our body image and self-concept.

- Help us develop and maintain friendships and relationships.

- Are needed to successfully carry on conversations, play games, and feel comfortable as part of a group.

- Are essential in obtaining and maintaining employment.

- Are lifelong skills necessary to be successful on the job and independent in adult life.

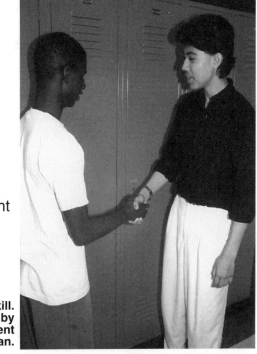

Greeting others is an important social skill. Shaking hands is a skill that is often learned by visual observation. Practice with the student whenever you can.

Why Teach Social Skills?

- Children typically learn play activities and other social interactions through visual observation and imitation. Students who are visually impaired often cannot observe and imitate others without instruction.

- Students with visual impairments often miss visual cues such as facial expressions and gestures. Consequently, they may have difficulty interpreting another person's feelings or actions.

- Sighted peers may interpret the visually impaired student's lack of eye contact, few facial expressions, and atypical body posture as disinterest, lack of concern, or simply strange.

- Students need opportunities to develop and practice social skills with different people in a variety of settings.

- Learning positive social skills will facilitate acceptance by classmates, employers, and others.

The Paraprofessional's Role

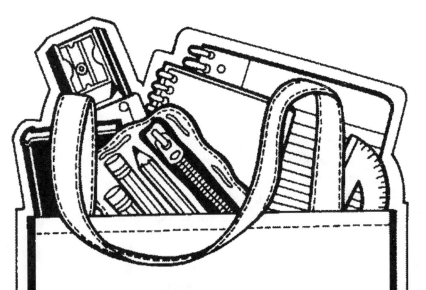

- **Because a paraprofessional may be with the student the most, you can make sure the student practices appropriate social skills.**

- **Help to implement and record progress on IEP objectives related to the student's social skills.**

- Work with students on specific activities which have been developed by the vision teacher to improve social skills.

- Participate in any available training which includes social skills development in students with visual impairments.

Suggestions

Here is a list of suggestions that may be helpful when you are working with your students. At the end of this chapter there are resources that can offer more suggestions for these areas.

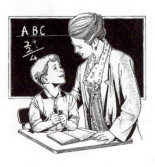

Body Language

- Explain to the students that people face each other when speaking. This behavior shows you are interested and paying attention to the person who is speaking. Encourage students to turn their body and direct their gaze toward the person speaking.

- Students with visual impairments may need opportunities to practice locating the approximate location of the face or voice of the person speaking.

- Provide opportunities to practice maintaining eye contact when speaking or listening to another in a variety of settings.

- Encourage appropriate body posture in sitting and standing positions, with head up in a natural and erect position. Pre-arranged signals such as an unobtrusive touch or special word can serve as reminders.

- Discuss facial expressions (e.g., happy, sad, angry) as feelings occur during the day. Encourage younger students to tactually and visually observe facial expressions. The use of mirrors, photographs, videos, and role playing can help build an understanding of facial expressions and gestures.

- Mannerisms such as rocking and eye-poking are often distracting or annoying to others. Provide the students with alternative activities such as rocking only in a rocking chair, or cradling forehead or side of head with a hand. In some cases, eyepoking can pose medical risks. The team may need to develop consistent strategies for decreasing unsafe mannerisms.

- Help the students develop an understanding and respect for personal physical space. During circle time students should keep their hands, feet, etc. to themselves. Other children may find it annoying for students with visual impairments to explore or touch them or their belongings.

- Through observation and role playing, students should learn to maintain appropriate physical space when talking to and working with others.

Classroom Skills

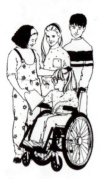

Note: These suggestions will be useful for students with verbal communication skills. Additional suggestions for students with multiple disabilities will be found in the chapter Students With Multiple Impairments on pages 127 to 152.

- At the beginning of the year, ask the vision teacher to educate the class about each student's visual impairment and its implications. Explain the use of special equipment and why materials, games, etc. may be adapted. Include students who are visually impaired if they would like to be involved, as appropriate.

- Encourage the students to communicate their visual needs and ask for help politely (e.g., "I cannot see the chart. May I move closer to look at it?").

- Demonstrate appropriate times to say "please", "thank you," "excuse me," etc.

- Students need to learn to interpret auditory and vocal cues. An example of an auditory cue might be when everyone stands to do the Pledge of Allegiance. Vocal cues help us understand when someone is angry, sad, etc.

- Activities which encourage turn-taking may include rolling a ball back and forth, talking on the telephone, simple card and board games, and computer games.

- Encourage the students to help their sighted peers, so they can experience being helpers, not just the one being helped by others.

- Model giving others compliments. Opportunities to practice this behavior can be provided through role play activities.

- Talk to the students about topics which are enjoyed by their peers such as current music, movies, toys, or styles in clothing. Provide concrete experiences to ensure understanding. This will help them learn what is *in* and they will be more able to join in conversations appropriately.

- Through listening and role playing, help the student learn how to approach his peers and initiate a conversation. (e.g., "Hi, how's it going?" or whatever is age-appropriate). This can be very intimidating to a child with limited vision. Practice helps build confidence.

- Provide activities and games which encourage conversational skills.

Cooperative Skills

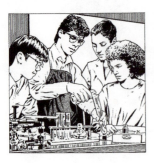

- Explain the rules of the classroom. Students who are visually impaired should be expected and encouraged to follow rules such as waiting quietly for their turn and raising their hand.

- Provide an environment that is structured and organized. Familiarize the students with learning centers and activities in those centers so they will know what to expect. Practice each activity to ensure understanding.

- Students with visual impairments may not observe or understand all of the activities in which their classmates are engaged. Describe activities that other students are doing. (e.g., "Sam and Ray are playing with toy cars." "Katie and Matt are building a castle with Lego™.") Check for understanding.

- Ask the vision teacher to make suggestions on how to adapt games that visually impaired students and their peers would enjoy playing (e.g., card games, board games). Explain the game rules to the student yourself rather than asking classmates. Give the students opportunities to learn and practice the game before playing it with their peers.

- Begin cooperative activities with small groups so there are frequent opportunities to practice.

Social Skills

- During recess or free play, provide toys for the students that would attract and interest their peers (e.g., action figures, electronic cars). To extend social interaction time with each other, provide activities such as jumping rope, tether ball, four square, and water or sand play.

- Select small groups to work or play in centers and change these combinations periodically. This enables students to learn more about everyone in the class.

- Avoid assigning someone to play with the student, as this may lead to resentment. Ask students with visual impairment for names of favorite classmates or solicit volunteers from the classmates. When selecting peers, choose those who will not try to take over or correct the student's efforts too frequently. Be available to monitor and guide the peers initially.

- Talk with the vision teacher, students, and their families about ways to socialize after school. Discuss social activities in the students' community such as scouts, going to the mall, bowling, skating, sports events, etc. Encourage the students to participate in some of these activities.

- Encourage the students to invite a friend to lunch, to play after school, to go to the park, etc. Discuss and provide practice through role play.

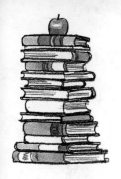

Additional Reading

The 1995-1996 guide to toys for children who are blind or visually impaired. New York: Joint Initiative of Toy Manufacturers of America and American Foundation for the Blind.

Kekelis, L., & Chernus-Mansfield, N. (1984). *Talk to me: A language guide for parents of blind children.* Los Angeles: Blind Children's Center.

Learning to play: Common concerns for the visually impaired preschool child. Los Angeles: Blind Children's Center.

Loumiet, R., & Levack, N. (1993). Introduction. In *Independent Living: A curriculum with adaptations for students with visual impairments. Vol. I. Social competence* (pp. 21-23). Austin, TX: Texas School for the Blind and Visually Impaired.

Meyers, L., & Lansky, P. (n. d.). *Dancing cheek to cheek.* Los Angeles: Blind Children's Center.

Welcome to the world: Toys and activities for the visually impaired infant. Los Angeles: Blind Children's Center.

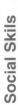

Social Skils

Daily Living Skills

by Nancy Levack & Cyral Miller

Paraprofessionals play an important role in helping students gain necessary daily living skills.

What Are Daily Living Skills?

Daily Living Skills address students' abilities to care for their personal needs, maintain personal health and safety, understand and carry out specific care related to their disability, and organize and maintain their personal environment.

The following categories address daily living skills activities that might be taught within a school program:

● Organizational Skills

● Self-Advocacy

● Personal Hygiene and Appearance

● Eating and Drinking

● Food Preparation

● Dressing and Clothing Care

● Health and Safety

Why Are They Important?

Daily Living Skills are important because they:

- Are lifelong skills which are critical throughout the students' lives.

- Have a huge impact on relationships.

- Develop independence.

- Make a significant difference in the level of care, quality of life, health and safety for students who have multiple disabilities.

- Impact vocational opportunities.

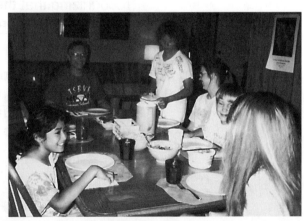

Eating and social skills are practiced at family dinners.

Why Teach Daily Living Skills?

- Students with visual impairments are at a distinct disadvantage in acquiring daily living skills since these skills are often learned through visual observation and imitation.

- Even low vision students who have a great deal of useful vision may miss many details about the procedures and refined movements needed to perform daily care tasks.

- People may assume students with visual impairments are not performing a particular daily living skill because they are not capable, instead of recognizing that their students may be able to successfully perform the tasks when instructed on how to do so.

- There are many specific procedures and adaptations which make these skills easier for a person who is visually impaired. Students should not be expected to discover these on their own.

The Paraprofessional's Role

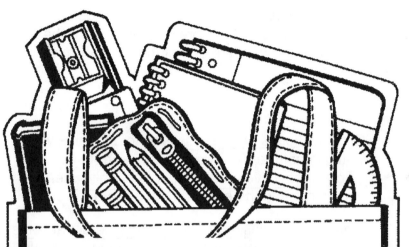

- The ARD committee will help determine priority areas for instruction. For these, there will be IEP goals written that you will help to implement and monitor for student progress.

- Discuss with parents and school staff what assistance the student requires and what is expected of the student in other daily living skills areas not addressed in the IEP.

- Be alert to signs of health problems. Often paraprofessionals are more closely involved with daily activities and can catch early signs of hygiene, eating, or health concerns. Communicating these back to the VI teacher, classroom teacher, and the parent can help the team develop and maintain appropriate goals.

Suggestions

Here is a list of practical suggestions that may be helpful when you are working with your students. Resources that can offer more suggestions for these areas can be found at the end of this chapter and in the Appendix.

Organizational Skills

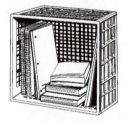

- Organization is an essential skill for students with visual impairments. Students can learn to be efficient, effective, and independent only when caregivers and the environment are organized.

- Material, supplies, and the student's personal items need to always be put back in the same place. Not only should students be shown where that place is, but they should be expected to get and return items independently as much as possible.

- Use a consistent and systematic approach when teaching a task (e.g., when entering the classroom, the student should learn a consistent routine that includes putting his coat and lunch in the same place).

- As students get older, they will need to learn how to take responsibility for their own organizational strategies.

- The more contained and defined a space is, the more organized a student can be. Drawer dividers, labels on shelves, containers, notebooks, and folders greatly add to organization.

Daily Living

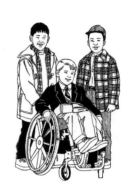

- There is a tendency to do too much for students. This is not helpful and it is a tremendous disservice to them because it makes the students seem more disabled than they are, isolates them from potential friends, and deprives them of learning the skills for themselves.

- Involve students as much as possible in deciding when help is needed and choosing an appropriate way or person to ask for that help.

- One way that help can be provided is to explain the environment to the student. There are times when a lack of vision limits the student's information about a situation. Someone who has more vision may need to describe the situation, give information about possible actions, and help the student problem solve a course of action.

- Students should be able to acknowledge when they can do things independently and may need to practice refusing assistance when they don't need help.

- Some students are afraid to make mistakes. Adults can help by creating a safe atmosphere for learning and practicing new skills. Often, students do not see others make mistakes and feel that they are the only ones who do so. It is helpful from time to time to point out if you have spilled something or broken something.

- A clear description of your job may help you, the student, and the student's peers to define what kind of help is needed and when.

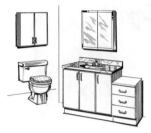

Personal Hygiene

Toileting and Hand Washing

- Students will need to be oriented to the location and arrangement of new bathrooms (e.g., where soap, sink, and towels are found).

- When accompanying or instructing students in a bathroom it is important to be aware of their right to privacy and use the least invasive approach needed to complete the task.

- Young students may need to be reminded about the importance of privacy and to close the door when toileting.

Toothbrushing

- Keep all toothbrushing items together and in the same place so they can be found easily.

- Students who have low vision can use a toothbrush and cup that visually contrast with each other and the sink or counter.

- Use tubes of toothpaste with flip tops or pump dispensers to prevent losing the small toothpaste cap.

- Students who have difficulty lining the toothpaste up on the toothbrush can squirt the toothpaste in their hand or tongue and then rub their toothbrush in the toothpaste before brushing.

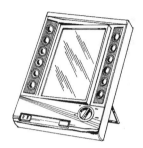

- Help students develop skills for reviewing their personal appearance.

- Some students who have low vision will benefit from mirrors that have lights and magnifiers.

- Electric shavers are safer and easier to use than razors.

- Clear nail polish gives a well groomed appearance and application mistakes are less noticeable.

- When students first learn how to apply makeup, they may need to practice blending it and asking for feedback from a person who can see to be sure that it is applied correctly.

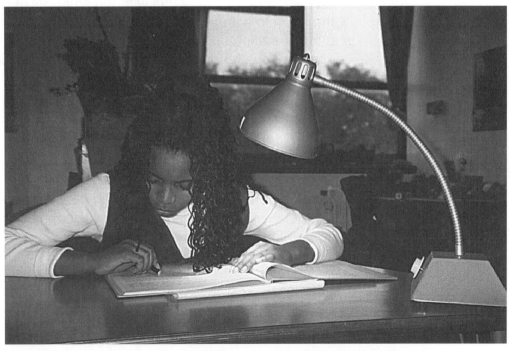

Students with visual impairments follow the same fashion trends as their peers. As a paraprofessional you may help them find "their look."

Daily Living

Eating and Drinking

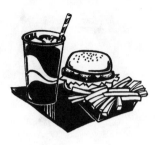

- Unbreakable dishes are very helpful when students are first learning how to eat.

- It is easier to see the food on dishes of contrasting color.

- Give young children the opportunity to play with dishes, utensils, and containers in water and sand. This gives them the opportunity to experiment with using these things at a time when messiness does not matter.

- One challenge when teaching eating skills is how to balance the need for direct instruction in natural contexts (e.g., the cafeteria) against the student's discomfort at being singled out among peers. It may be helpful to negotiate this with the students and/or the team to set up some guidelines. Some options may be setting up private instruction, agreeing on specific days for cafeteria instruction, or setting up unobtrusive signals between students and staff members when help is needed.

- Students can be taught to request information about what is being put on the tray as they go through the serving line.

- When teaching scooping, start with heavier foods like mashed potatoes so the students can tell when something is on the spoon.

- Students may need to be taught a subtle but effective way to touch their food in order to tell what is on their plate.

- Using the fork to scrape the food towards the center of the plate increases the likelihood of getting something and reduces the chances of food spilling off the edge of the plate.

- Cutting with a knife is one of the most difficult eating skills. Some tips that can make the task easier are using a serrated knife, lining up the knife along the back of the fork to cut, using the width of the tines of the fork to estimate a bite size piece, and setting the knife across the top of the plate with the cutting edge consistently facing the center of the plate.

- Teach students to use a consistent pattern for spreading (e.g., edge to edge, putting food in the center and radiating out).

- Some students may want to review the school menu and choose to bring a packed lunch when a food is being served that is particularly difficult to eat.

- A common method of locating food is to imagine the plate as a clock face with food at specific hours, such as potatoes at 9 o'clock and corn at 2 o'clock. The plate can be turned so that the meat is at 6 o'clock for ease of locating and cutting. Another option is to place the best anchored food, such as mashed potatoes, at 11 o'clock (2 o'clock for left handed eaters) so that harder to manage foods such as peas can be scooped up against the denser food.

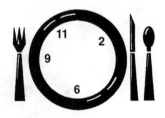

- When a plate of food is served, students can ask peers where the food is located on the plate and use a fork to feel for it, distinguishing the difference in consistency and texture.

- When using salt and pepper it is helpful to shake them into the hand and then shake them on to the food to get a more accurate amount.

- When pouring from a carton into a glass, it is helpful to hold the glass and carton so that hands are opposite each other, tilt the carton towards the glass and slide the glass upward against the side of the carton until the rim of the glass is under the spout. As the glass fills, the pouring sound and the changing temperature of the glass are added clues for when to stop.

- Another method for pouring is to put one finger over the edge of the glass or cup and stop pouring when the liquid touches the finger tip. Obviously, this does not work as well with hot liquids!

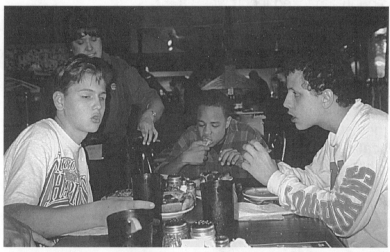

Eating out lets the students practice their social, orientation and mobility, and eating skills. Here students discuss topics about Italy while eating pizza.

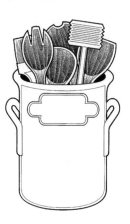

Food Preparation

- Organization is important in any type of food preparation. Some tricks may include using trays as work areas to define a work space, always putting things back in the same place so they can be found again, and using a simple labeling system on shelves and items.

- There is a lot of adaptive equipment that makes cooking easier (e.g. timers, cutting guides, liquid level indicators, lock lid pots, large print measuring devices). Catalogs can be ordered from the list of suppliers in the Appendix on pages 154 to 155.

- Teach students to use a systematic approach for cleaning a table or counter.

- When stirring, use long handled spoons and large bowls to prevent spills.

- When cooking, extra long kitchen mitts can prevent burns on arms and hands.

Daily Living

Dressing and Clothing Care

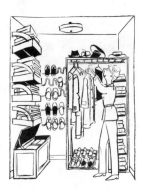

- When teaching dressing skills to young children, it is helpful to stand behind them and use hand-over-hand assistance to guide the natural movement.

- It may take more time and practice for children who are visually impaired to dress, but the reward in self-esteem and increased independence is worth the effort.

- Students may need to be taught about privacy. One way to reinforce the right to privacy is by asking permission or giving notice before helping a student to undress.

- A systematic approach to storing clothing can help both at school and at home (e.g., hanging jackets in the same place).

- Initially, hand clothing to a student the same way each time. In time, teach the parts of clothing and how to turn them around so they are in the correct position for putting on.

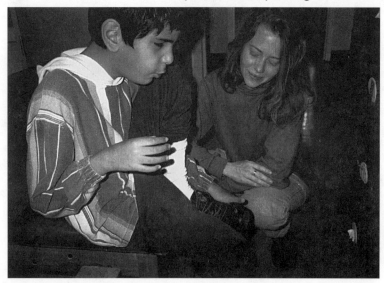

- There are many ways that clothing can be labeled, including placing small safety pins or buttons in a certain place and using aluminum braille labels.

Give the student a chance to manage on his own before physically helping him. This residential instructor waits for the student's request to tie his shoes.

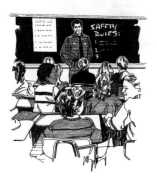

- Get information from the vision teacher about the reason for the students' visual impairments. Ask if there is anything related to health or safety that you need to be aware of. For example, if a student has glaucoma, you may be asked to watch for signs of headache or eye pain.

- Arrange a secret signal such as an unobtrusive special word or touch, that can serve as a reminder to a student to sit or stand up straight or to control mannerisms such as eyepoking. The team may need to work together to develop effective strategies to address very persistent mannerisms.

- Ask the orientation and mobility instructor to help you and the students plan safe ways to travel and move within the school environment.

- Involve students in problem solving how to safely participate in activities.

- Review safety routines for fire drills with the teacher and the student so that the student is prepared.

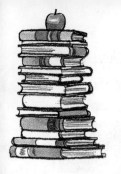

Additional Reading

Brody, J., & Webber, L. (1994). *Let's eat: Feeding a child with a visual impairment.* Los Angeles: Blind Children's Center.

Condon, R. (1992). *Toilet training children with deaf/blindness/multiple disabilities: Issues and strategies.* Unpublished handout. (Available from Outreach Department Texas School for the Blind and Visually Impaired, 1100 West 45th St., Austin, TX 78756-3494.)

Ferrell, K. A. (1985). Coming across: Daily living and communicating. *Reach out and teach: meeting training needs of parents of visually and multiply handicapped young children* (pp. 141-172). New York: American Foundation for the Blind.

Loumiet, R., & Levack, N. (1993). *Independent living: A curriculum with adaptations for students with visual impairments. Vol. II Self-care and maintenance of personal environment.* 2nd ed. Austin: Texas School for the Blind and Visually Impaired.

Mangold, P. N. (1980). *The pleasures of eating for those who are visually impaired.* Castro Valley, CA: Exceptional Teaching Aids.

Swallow, R. M., & Huebner, K. M. (1987). *How to thrive, not just survive: A guide to developing independent living skills for blind and visually impaired children and youths.* New York: American Foundation for the Blind.

Daily Living

Orientation and Mobility Skills

by Sharon Trusty and Olga Uriegas

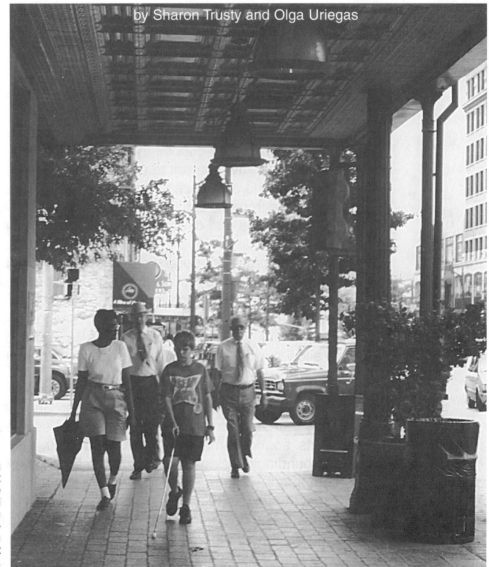

Helping a student experience the world around him and gain self-confidence in independent travel.

What Are Orientation and Mobility Skills?

How do people know where they are, where they want to go and how to get to their destinations? Most people automatically look around to recognize where they are, then they choose the best way to move through the environment to arrive at their destination and avoid the obstacles in their way. Their vision instantly combines colors, shapes, and movements with memories and directions into information they can use to travel safely and efficiently. Often, this process is so automatic that people can tell by looking if they are moving in the direction they need to go. These skills are orientation and mobility (O&M) skills. They are learned by experience and by observing others. The mental, visual and movement skills work together to allow people to move easily in any environment.

Orientation is the process people use to detect where they are and where objects are around them. They gather information with their senses such as sights, sounds, smells and textures of their surroundings. Using directions and memories, people compare the information they receive to what they expect to find. In this way, people can identify where they are and decide if that is where they need to be, then move to their destinations.

Mobility is the physical movement of the person from one place to another. Mobility and movement skills begin when babies crawl to favorite toys. As children learn more complex skills, they will learn to walk, skip, run, and ride bicycles.

Orientation and mobility (O&M) assessments are completed by O&M specialists certified by the Association for Education and Rehabilitation of the Blind and Visually Impaired (AER). Assessment areas for all students with visual impairments include concepts about body, space, and movement, as well as how the students move around their classrooms, schools, and neighborhoods. Information on how directions are remembered and followed is important for the O&M instructor to know. If the students can see, how well they see colors, shapes, objects, and movements will be important as they learn to travel independently.

Why are Orientation and Mobility Skills Important?

O&M skills are used by people with visual impairments to make their travel safe, confident, responsible and independent. These skills enable people with visual impairments and blindness to travel in any environment, whether or not it is familiar to them.

Success in mobility is associated with a good self-concept as a person with a visual impairment. Efficient travel skills help develop problem-solving abilities. Vocational success may depend on the ability to travel independently. To arrive on time to classes or appointments, people who are blind or visually impaired must choose correct and timely routes and transportation.

Movement is critical to physical well-being. With O&M skills, students with visual impairments can try out a variety of exercise options and choose those that best meet their needs. Movement can reduce stress and encourage good health.

When students cannot see what is ahead of them, one of the greatest risks they may take is to move from where they feel *safe*. They may become lost if they have not spent time learning the names and shapes of objects in the area, or in practicing moving from one place to another. Students with visual impairments who have had unfortunate experiences or accidents may need to relearn or learn modified skills.

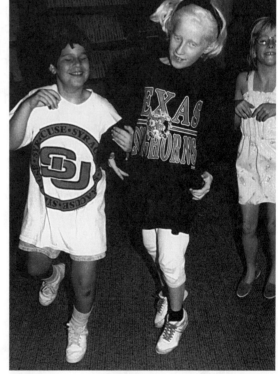

**Joy in movement!
Experiencing movement in space in a
safe environment increases self-
awareness and exercises the body.**

Why Teach Orientation and Mobility Skills?

When students have no vision, unreliable vision, or limitations in vision, they need to be shown specific techniques and ways to learn about their environments. They must be taught strategies to use the information from their other senses to know where they are and where they want to go. People who cannot see can move safely if instruction is provided in using different techniques. These travel techniques are not commonly known and cannot be learned without direct intervention. For example:

● Protective arm techniques

● Trailing

● Sighted guide

● Use of adaptive mobility devices

Using an adaptive mobility (pre-cane) device that is designed to detect drop-offs. This bumper cane is made of PVC pipes by the O&M instructor.

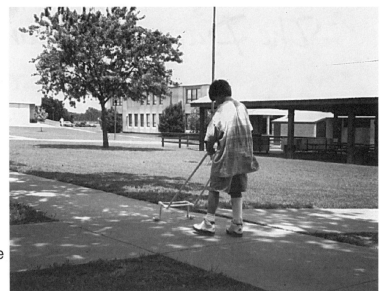

To be able to use these traveling techniques, students start by moving around and exploring objects. They must learn the names of objects and the parts of their bodies. They are taught to use the information from sounds and textures to orient themselves in sensory training activities. These skills work together to help the students move safely and efficiently to their destinations.

Family members and people who work with these students may unintentionally limit movements because of safety concerns. Learning and practicing basic safety rules under the guidance of an O&M instructor makes the student a safer traveler.

These safety rules, such as keeping to the right and waiting at the corner for traffic to pass before crossing the street, are typically observed and then reinforced by watching what others do. Students with visual impairments will need more direct instruction and reinforcement to master efficient and safe travel.

Orientation & Mobility

The Paraprofessional's Role

The paraprofessional supports and reinforces the instruction that is planned and carried out by the O&M instructor. It is up to the O&M instructor to assess the students, determine their needs, provide instruction and train the staff members who work with the students. The paraprofessional will need direct instruction from the O&M instructor on specific techniques such as sighted guide. Since students need to practice their orientation and mobility skills in all environments, the support of the families and other school staff members will be important to the progress of the student.

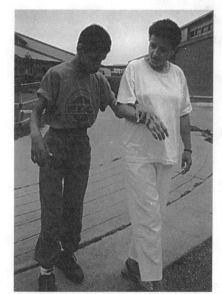

The time the students spend with the O&M instructor may not be long enough for the O&M instructor to see all the strengths and challenges of the students. The skills the students show may vary during the day and during the week. It will be the paraprofessional's role to communicate observations back to the O&M instructor so that the O&M instructor can make informed decisions about the students' programs.

An adapted sighted guide technique is used when the student is not steady enough using a conventional sighted guide technique.

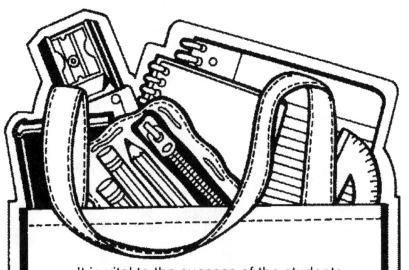

It is vital to the success of the students that the paraprofessional knows:

- The techniques that the students are learning

- Why the students are learning these techniques

- The ways in which the students can be corrected

- The progress the students make

- Areas where the students have difficulties during the day.

Suggestions

Concepts

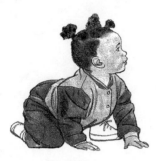

Many young children with visual impairments and blindness have not had the same experiences as other children of the same age. This may be due to medical conditions and treatments, protectiveness of the people who cared for them, or simply lack of opportunity to visually observe and learn from objects or environments around them. Active intervention is needed to increase their grasp of basic concepts.

• Orientation skills begin with movement and exploration. Babies who cannot see do not realize that the sounds they like to hear are rattles or toys moving back and forth. The babies who cannot see have no way to connect sounds to any type of motion unless they hold and move the toys.

• Allowing young children many opportunities to explore a variety of objects is important. They can learn that their movements cause objects to make sounds. As children explore their world with guided assistance, they will learn the names, qualities, and characteristics of the objects. This will give the students an understanding of what is in their environment.

- Without vision, learning about objects and the use of objects will be different from most people's experience. Children with visual impairments will need to use touch. They may not be able to see objects as a whole. They may need to build a whole concept of an object from the parts that they can feel, hear, taste and smell. If an object makes sound, bring the object and the child together to demonstrate that the sound is coming from that specific source. When children are using touch and sound to gain information about objects, learning may take longer, especially when the objects become more complex.

- The students must learn the purposes and functions of objects around them in their own ways since they cannot glance over and see what others are doing with the objects. Skills for examining objects with their hands may need to be demonstrated and discussed. Discussion can help students remember what they know from their experiences and apply that information to what they are learning.

- Directional concepts help students understand actions and locations of objects. As others try to help the students find things or places, it is important that the students understand the words used so they can follow the directions given to them. The students must learn to use words like *right, left, faster, slower, upper* and *lower*. Guided practice in use of these terms must be provided.

- When describing objects, add the qualities or characteristics of the objects such as colors, textures, shapes and sizes. These qualities help the students in classifying and comparing objects. These terms must be taught as they are introduced to the students.

- Make sure the language used describes what the child is experiencing.

- Stronger concepts are built when students actively interact with their world instead of simply hearing and talking about it.

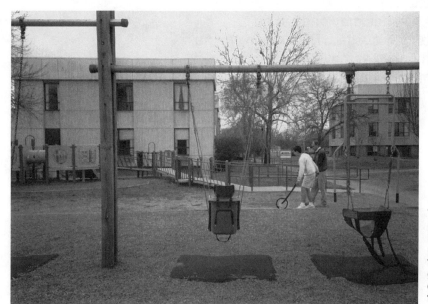

This student and instructor are measuring a playground with a trundle wheel that gives an audible click for every foot measured.

Students begin to understand how they move when they know the names and locations of their body parts and how they work together. As students learn how their bodies can move, they develop coordination. Once the students understand how their bodies work, they can connect this knowledge to moving in their immediate environments. Later, the children will learn that the movement and characteristics they experienced are similar to those experiences by other people.

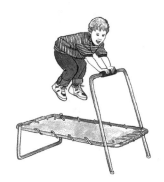

- An understanding of body image contributes to the development of good posture. Good posture is important for the body to function properly. It will enable the students with visual impairments to move and use their other senses more easily. Good posture can also help persons with visual impairments to blend in with groups, which will strengthen positive self-concepts. Poor posture can attract unnecessary attention to the students, setting them apart from others in their classes. Often it helps to develop a pre-arranged signal to unobtrusively remind students to maintain good posture.

- There are specific techniques students can use to detect objects while moving. Young students use protective arm technique to do this. Students need to understand where their arms are in relation to their bodies and that holding their arms in this position will protect them from getting hurt by detecting obstacles. As students move safely in their environments, they will gain confidence and experience.

Sensory Training

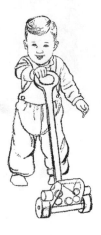

Early opportunities for exploration and experimentation are vital for children. Students with no vision must rely on their other senses to put sounds, feelings, sensations and words together. Students will move with more ease in their environments when they recognize cues and use their senses to discriminate differences.

• Students who cannot see must rely on remembered sounds and feelings for information that helps them know where they are. Young children may find where their parents are from the sound of water splashing in the sink, the scent from the coffeepot, the cool tile of the floor, or the hum of the refrigerator. It will be important for students to find and identify landmarks within the school environment that will help them know where they are.

• Students who are visually impaired rely heavily on using their hands to gain information. Avoid forcing their hands into unpleasant or unfamiliar experiences without careful preparation and the student's consent.

- Children with visual impairments may be reluctant or unwilling to touch unfamiliar objects as a way of protecting themselves from too much information or from an unpleasant or painful sensory experience. This sensitivity, called tactual defensiveness, may prevent the children from getting all the information from the environment that they need. Since much of the information the children learn will be from touch, this defensiveness must be addressed. For example, a child may need a gradual introduction to other textures similar to the way that babies are introduced to new foods. Sometimes it is helpful if new textures are paired with familiar items. It is very important that the educational team addresses this issue and develops specific strategies for the individual. An occupational therapist may be a very helpful resource.

- Children with visual impairments may prefer to play with real objects and nontraditional toys. Many traditional toys for young children are made of the same type of plastic, are tactually uninteresting, and have only visual differences.

- It is important for students to use vision and other senses for independent travel. Listening to a person tapping on a table may be a good cue for moving to it.

Motor Development

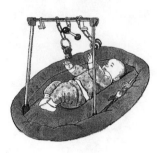

Motor development for children with visual impairments may be delayed or slower than for other children. Students who cannot see to move toward interesting objects miss the movement practice that other children have. Often the children have additional impairments which make motor skills development more difficult. Students with visual impairments will need specific learning experiences to develop the necessary strength and balance to move in a normal way.

- When infants with visual impairment are learning to roll over, having them roll toward something is more motivating than simply rolling with no purpose. Reaching to an object or light when on their sides will help them learn to use their bodies for a purpose.

- Skills such as reaching across midline to learn to roll over onto their stomach may have to be taught so that students can learn the skills needed for crawling (e.g., positioning desirable objects across the child's midline and helping the child reach for the objects).

- Movement experiences should be positive and successful so that students are not afraid to move.

- Rehearsing skills mentally and verbally can help some students learn faster and remember the skill longer.

- Avoid meaningless practice. Use movement in a functional manner to get somewhere important (e.g., recess, a drink).

- Students with visual impairments may need tactual and auditory cues rather than visual cues as they learn to move in their environments. Look for naturally occurring cues (e.g., the end of a hallway, a water fountain motor, doorways, changes in floor texture) to help students move in their classroom, school or home. Increasing visual/tactual contrast will help students locate their own locker in the hallway.

Techniques are taught by the O&M specialist and reinforced by others based on information from evaluation of the skills of the students, travel needs of the students, and the environments the students will be using. Consult with the O&M instructor to know how to implement these strategies.

Rolling Canes, Adaptive Canes, and Push Toys

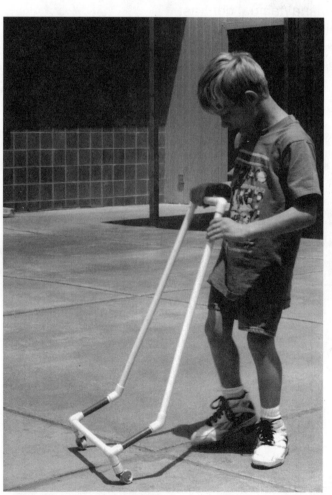

Young children use push toys or adapted canes (e.g., rolling) in front of them for stability and to run into obstacles near the ground that their hands might not encounter. As the toy or cane bumps into an obstacle, they can move it toward the obstacle, take a step to the side, and move the toy forward until the obstacle is no longer being bumped. In this way, the children can continue to walk in the same direction as they started.

This rolling cane (the Wheeler) adds stability when running into obstacles.

Protective Arm Techniques

To protect the upper body, one arm is bent at the elbow and held up across the body at shoulder level with the palm facing out. This helps to detect objects at head and chest level. To protect the lower abdomen, the other arm is fully extended down the center of the lower abdomen with the palm toward the body. These techniques are used in familiar areas for short periods. This angle allows the hand to contact objects first, resulting in a maximum reaction time.

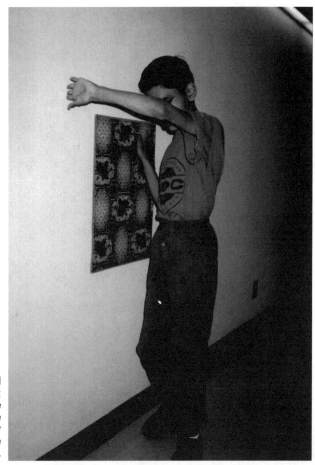

A carpet sample stapled to the wall serves as an artificial landmark; this student gets the cue to square off to the classroom door on the opposite side. This is also a very good demonstration of protective forearm technique.

Orientation & Mobility

Trailing

Trailing is a technique used indoors on familiar routes to travel in a straight line. Facing the direction of travel the student stands with the side of the body toward the object used for trailing (e.g., wall); then extends the arm nearest the wall with the palm down and fingers flexed in toward the palm. The student puts the ring or little finger lightly against the wall and moves forward. In hallways, trailing should be on the right side to move with the flow of traffic.

The other arm can be held in a protective arm position to protect the body, depending on the height of the obstacles that will be encountered. If trailing the school hall, the upper body position will help detect doors or lockers that are partially open while the hand that is trailing the wall will detect objects near the lower body.

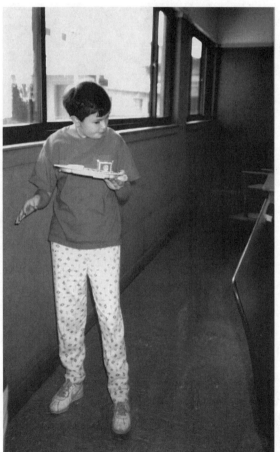

This student is putting her little finger lightly against the wall to trail in the cafeter.

Orientation & Mobility

Sighted Guide

The sighted guide technique is the easiest way for students with visual impairments to walk with a person who can see. The guide should touch the student's arm to signal the student, and allow the student's hand to move up to grasp the guide's arm above the elbow. The student should hold onto the guide's arm with the thumb outside the guide's arm and the fingers inside the guide's arm. The student can hold the arm bent at the elbow and close to the body while holding onto the guide's arm. This position will put the student about one-half step behind the guide, providing the guide a clear view to each side for safe travel. It will also give the students a short time to react as the guide stops, turns, or steps up or down. The guide should walk at a normal pace, slowing for younger children. As the guide approaches a step up or down, he should slow to signal to the student that a change is coming up. To end the grip, the guide should turn his arm out as he turns his body toward the student. The student should let go of the guide's arm.

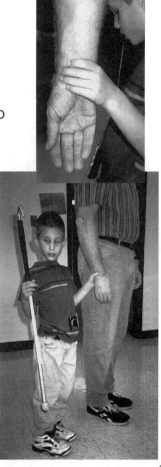

Wrist method for sighted guide technique

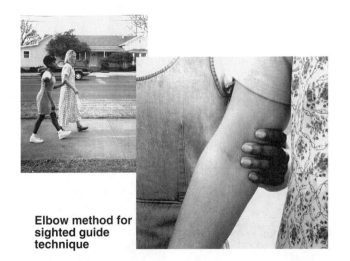

Elbow method for sighted guide technique

Seating

When helping seat students, the guide should lead the student near the seat. The guide will tell the student where the chair is in relation to the student. The student should let go of the guide's arm and move one foot to contact the chair leg. The student can hold up an arm to protect the face. The other hand should sweep across the chair seat to clear the chair and see how it is facing. The student can turn around to line up the back of his legs with the front edge of the chair and seat himself. When rising, the guide can stand beside the student and contact the student's arm to get into position to guide.

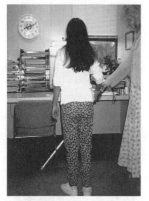

1. Approaching the chair

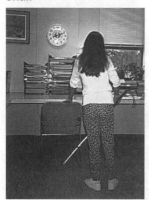

2. Locating back of chair

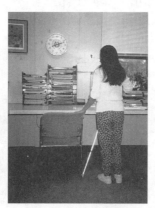

3. Cane locates side of chair

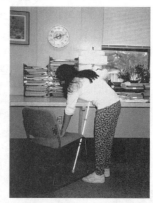

4. Clearing seat of chair

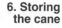

6. Storing the cane

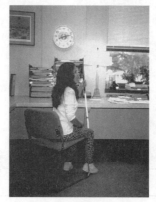

5. Line up back of legs with front of seat before sitting down

Room Familiarization

One of the most important aspects of room familiarization is allowing students to spend time being oriented to the objects of the room. In this way students will learn how the room is constructed. Starting at the door, the guide can walk with the student clockwise around the perimeter of the classroom to give the student an idea of the size of the room. The next walk around the room could be exploration of the objects found along the wall including the chalkboard, bulletin board, pencil sharpeners, windows, closets, lockers, etc. The student could then travel around the room independently by trailing the walls or book shelves, name the objects encountered, and ask questions about the objects not recognized. Encourage systematic exploration of all parts of the room.

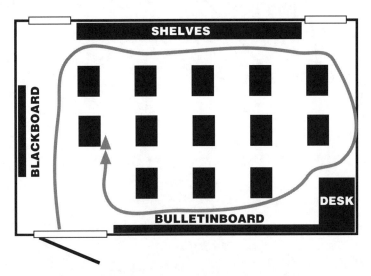

Starting at the door the guide can walk with the student clockwise around the perimeter of the classroom to give the student an idea of the size of the room.

Recovering Dropped Objects

The student should face in the direction of the sound the object made as it lands on the floor. The student should move toward the sound using protective arm techniques to protect the face when bending down or kneeling near where the sound was.

There are two ways the students can move their hands flat on the ground to find the object: the circular pattern and the grid pattern. The circular pattern is simply moving the hand in small circles on the floor until the dropped object is found. The grid pattern starts at the knee or the foot. The students will move their hands from the knee out, then back and forth alongside the knee to find the object. They can then move their hands to the right or left and use the same back and forth movements. If the item is not found, they move a step forward and repeat the movement.

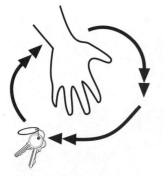

Circular search pattern

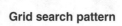

Grid search pattern

Using the Long Cane

Some students will be instructed in the use of the long cane by the O&M instructor. For the diagonal technique, the cane is held in one position diagonally in front of the body. Touch technique is more complicated and requires constant motion of the hand holding the cane to detect drop-offs and objects. As with other specific O&M techniques, close coordination with the instructor, classroom teachers and parents is needed to ensure proper practice throughout the day.

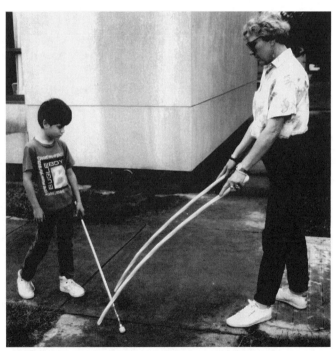

Teaching touch technique with an arc definer helps to get the feel for the width of the sweeping movement.

Activities

The paraprofessional reinforces the skills taught by the O&M instructor. Some suggested activities follow. The O&M instructor should be consulted to confirm that the activities are appropriate to meet individual needs.

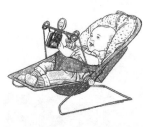

For infants and toddlers:

- For sound awareness, make sounds with an object and let the child touch it as it makes sounds.

- When the child reaches for an object consistently, move the object a little farther away to increase movement.

- Leave sound toys next to the child so that his arm and leg movements create sounds.

- Describe and imitate sounds that are *fast, high, loud, low, slow, and soft.*

- When changing the child's clothing, tell him what you are doing. Name the parts of the body as he gets dressed.

- Allow the child to feel objects that are *coarse, fine, damp, dry, soft, hard, heavy, light, smooth, rough, hot, cold, warm, cool, sharp, blunt, slippery, slimy,* and *slick* and name the textures he touches.

- Use words that describe where objects are in relation to the child: *over, under, around, through.*

For elementary students:

- Identify indoor and outdoor sounds when walking to different locations during the day.

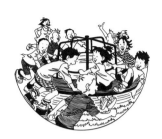

- To practice localizing sounds, ask the student to walk toward voices, handclaps, etc.

- When working with the student, look for ways to introduce and reinforce body, spatial, and environmental concepts.

- Allow the student to explore his classroom(s). In a familiar area, have him find a specific sound in the room.

- As the student walks, ask him to describe how the surface feels. A distinct change in the texture of the walking surface can serve as a landmark to help find locations.

- Walk around the edge of the playground, using the fence and the terrain to learn about the area.

- Give directions that use the terms *right* and *left* in routes and in games.

- When giving directions, use measurements such as *distances* (e.g., inch, foot, yard, block, mile) and *time* (e.g., second, minute, hours, morning, noon, afternoon, evening, night). Use real objects as students are learning measurement (e.g., how many steps to cross a room compared to going down the hall).

- The students will need to know how to climb, crawl, jump, pivot, tiptoe, gallop, leap, slide, skip, swing, march, dodge, roll, run, and walk. They will also need to use their bodies to beckon, bend, bounce, clap, fall, jump, kneel, lift, nod "yes" and "no," pout, relax, shake, shrug, squat, stretch, twist or turn, wave, wink. Play games using these directions to practice and increase understanding.

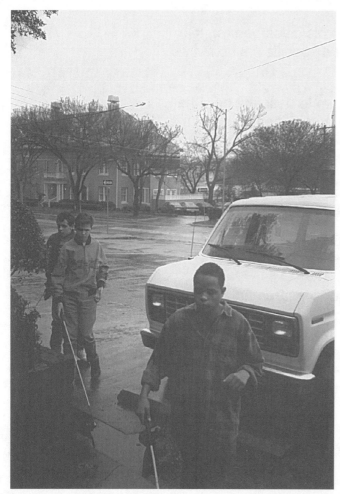

Manuevering safely around obstacles in unfamiliar areas

Additional Reading

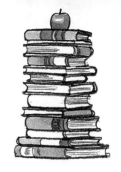

Dodson-Burk, B., & Hill, E. W. (1989). *An orientation and mobility primer for families and young children.* New York: American Foundation for the Blind.

Move with me: A parent's guide to movement development for visually impaired babies. Los Angeles: Blind Children's Center.

Simmons, S. S., & Maida, S. O. (n. d.). *Reaching, crawling, walking.... let's get moving: Orientation and mobility for preschool children.* Los Angeles: Blind Children's Center.

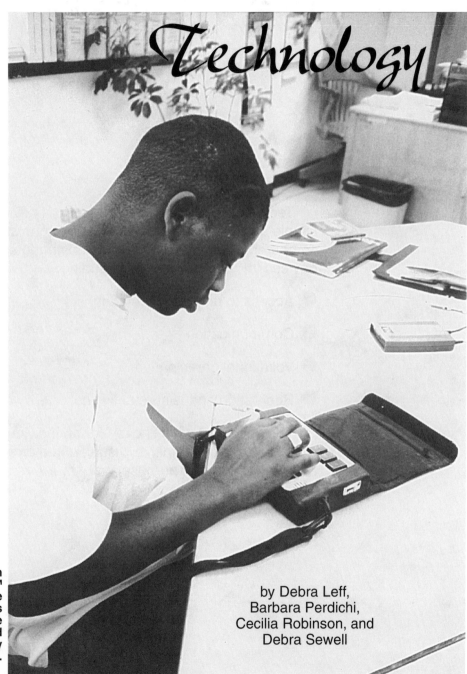

Technology

Taking notes with a Braille-Lite™ with refreshable braille output lets students store their notes and print to any printing device.

by Debra Leff,
Barbara Perdichi,
Cecilia Robinson, and
Debra Sewell

What Is Technology?

Technology can be used to refer to a device as simple as a switch or as complex and sophisticated as computers. Students with visual impairments may use devices for many purposes, including:

● Access to printed information

● Communication

● Vocational participation

● Recreation and leisure activities

The specific device chosen for an individual student will depend upon cognitive, visual, and motor abilities, and the educational purpose.

Why Is It Important?

- Many kinds of technology tools are now available which can maximize participation in learning and school routines.

- Technology is one of many tools used to enhance students' educational programs. Technological expertise can be a determining factor in adult vocational success.

- Increasingly, technology can also create opportunities for satisfying leisure pursuits.

- A technology tool for self-organization and self-management increases independence and self-reliance.

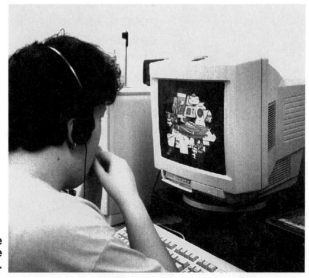

Games make students comfortable with computers and can enhance their visual functioning.

Technology

Why Teach Technology?

The federal IDEA law says that children with disabilities must be provided supplementary services that permit them to benefit from their education. Technology support is considered a supplementary service. For many students with visual impairments, technology is an essential tool for independence.

Computers are becoming commonplace even in classrooms for very young children. In addition, touch screens, alternative keyboards, switches, large print and speech software are widely used for students with visual and other impairments. However, students may need modifications in order to make typical technology devices or computer programs accessible to them. They need instruction to use modifications in addition to learning computer and other concepts offered in regular programs. Other modifications, such as lighting or positioning, as well as unique considerations for students with visual impairments, will require the expertise of the vision teacher.

Technology

Changes in Technology

Technology changes at a rapid rate. It is almost impossible for anyone to keep up with its pace. For students with visual impairments, access to technology is always going to be a challenge. Modifications may be necessary to meet the unique needs of these students. There is a variety of equipment, devices, and programs currently used by students with visual impairments. Even though more sophisticated devices and programs are available, they may or may not be appropriate for your student. When you are in doubt and feel that a change in the student's technology is needed, talk to the vision teacher so that your concerns or comments can be brought to the student's IEP team.

Technology

The Paraprofessional's Role

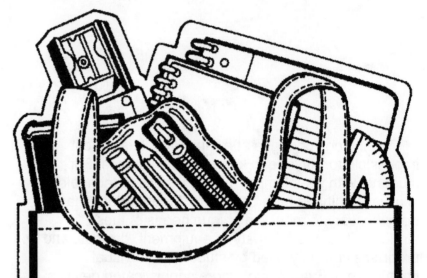

- Your goal is to carry out the student's technology objectives, and work with the students on the activities that have been assigned. You should work with the vision teacher to develop strategies that empower students to develop their skills.

- It would be beneficial to participate in technology training suitable to the needs of the students with whom you are working. Talk with the vision teacher about obtaining necessary training.

- You may also help the students maintain their equipment and obtain repairs or replacements as needed.

Suggestions

- Encourage the student to sit up while using devices. Reading stands or stands mounted to the side of the computer monitor facilitate good posture.

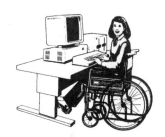

- Make sure that tables and chairs are at the appropriate height for each student. The student's arms should be at her side when writing or typing, and feet should touch the floor.

- The closed circuit television and computer monitors should be placed at the student's eye level. They may need to be moved closer or further from the student for best viewing.

*Placement of
Device*

- The switch, communication device, notetaker, or keyboard can be placed on the table or on the student's lap or lap tray. When necessary, they can be secured by tape or *Velcro™*.

- Some devices can be mounted on a wheelchair or on a slanted surface. Ensure comfort and accessibility.

Technology

Using Technology Tools

- When compared to their sighted peers, students with visual impairments probably have more concepts to learn when using technology devices. Help students learn these concepts in a systematic manner. Concrete and honest feedback on their performance may be helpful.

- Allow students enough time to learn and use their devices. Technology is intended to increase their independence.

- Help students come up with and use an alternative method to complete a task when technology fails. For example, a blind student should use a braille writer to do his work when the braille notetaker fails.

- Remember that technology is a tool that enables students to participate in or complete a task. It is not an end in itself. Look at the activity that the student is being asked to complete. Determine how technology will facilitate this task. Technology needs to be taught for a designated purpose.

Information About Different Kinds of Technology

The areas of technology addressed in this handbook include:

- Switches

- Augmentative Communication Devices

- Alternative Keyboards

- Enlarging Systems/Devices

- Tactual Graphics

- Notetaking Devices

- Reference Systems

- Computer Systems

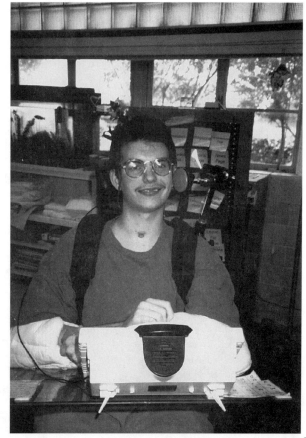

Technology is for everyone. This student can operate a Dynavox (communication device) with a headswitch mounted on his wheelchair.

Technology

Switches

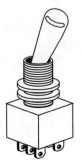

Switches can either be plugged directly into a device or can be plugged into a control unit with a timer. They can be accessed from a variety of positions depending on the student's motor skills. Switches allow increased environmental accessibility and can be created from a variety of materials (Rocklage, et al).

Types of Switches

pressure-sensitive
  (e.g., pillow)
movement-sensitive
  (e.g., air)
button
lever
rocker

Use to Teach

cause and effect
choice-making
requesting
turn-taking
commenting
participation in activities

Sample Activities

snack-making
music activities
recreation/leisure activities
computer games
group participation/games
writing in Morse code

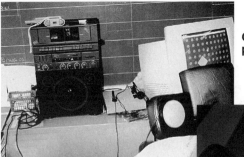

Operating a radio/cassette player with a headswitch

The student can be involved in stapling paper together by hooking up a switch to an electric stapler.

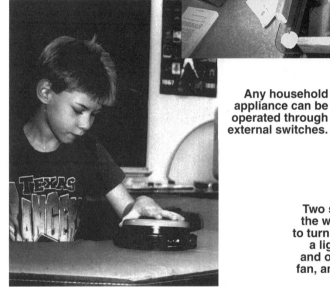

Any household appliance can be operated through external switches.

Two switches on the wall are used to turn a radio and a light chain on and off, control a fan, and make the bed move.

A Big Mac™ switch allows the student to communicate by listening to instruction or a phrase recorded by the teacher. The student can also record a phrase of his own.

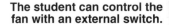

The student can control the fan with an external switch.

Augmentative Communication Devices

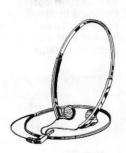

Voice output devices can be programmed to meet specific student needs. Some of these are appropriate for the student with basic communication needs, while others are used to support the student with multiple impairments in the academic setting.

There are many of these devices on the market and they change quickly due to advances in technology. In general, voice output devices can have digitized or synthetic speech. Digitized speech sounds more like a human voice whereas synthesized speech is more robotic. Some of the devices are stand-alone systems while others can be used with a computer.

To become an effective communication partner, appropriate training and support is necessary when using augmentative communication devices.

Communication Devices*	Digitized Speech	Synthetic Speech	Stand-Alone	Computer Based
Wolf®	●		●	●
Alpha Talker®	●		●	
Walker Talker®	●		●	
Liberator®	●		●	●
Speak Easy®	●		●	
Intro Talker®	●		●	
Power Pad®		●		●
IntelliKeys[1]®	●	●		●
Delta Talker®	●		●	
Dynavox®	●	●		
Big Mac®	●	●		
Cheap Talk 4[2]®	●		●	
Macaw®	●		●	
DAC®	●		●	

[1]used with Overlay Maker
[2]switch module

*This list of devices is subject to change depending upon technological advances.

Technology

Use to Teach

choice-making

requesting

commenting

sequencing of events

reporting

giving instructions or comments

participating in group activities

Sample activities

reinforcing academic skills

giving directions during cooking activity

participating in fingerplays/songs/ poetry

commenting on the day's activities

delivering messages (lunch count, attendance, courier)

1 Alpha Talker®
2 Using a Macaw® in his lap to give instructions to other students in a cooking activity
3 DAC®
4 IntelliKeys® with a Macintosh®

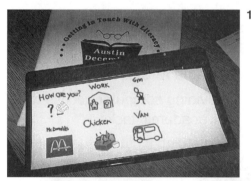

1

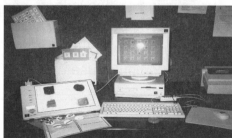

2

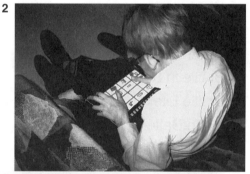

3

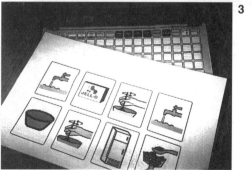

4

Technology

Alternative Keyboards

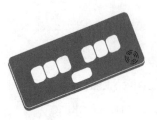

Alternative keyboards are used for students who cannot access a standard computer keyboard. Some of these are appropriate for the student with basic communication needs, while others are used to support the student with multiple impairments in the academic setting. They give students who are physically challenged an alternative access system for the computer.

Keyboards*

Unicorn® board

IntelliKeys®

Key Largo®

TASH®

TASH Mini®

Power Pad®

Big Keys®

BAT Personal Keyboard[1]®

Braille 'n Speak[1]®

Braille Lite[1]®

MountBatten Brailler[1]®

[1]Keyboards for one-handed users available

Uses for Keyboards

concept development

basic communication

picture and tactual discrimination

beginning literacy/number identification

Sample Activities

providing computer access for academic tasks

reinforcing picture or tactual symbols

playing games to learn early computer literacy skills

integrating motor skills with computer use

Technology

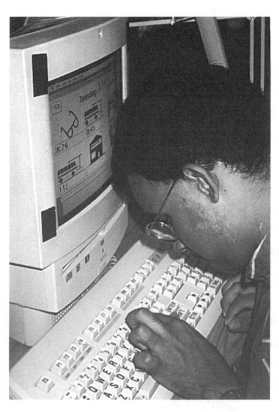

A conventional keyboard with large visible letters lets this student create his daily activities calendar.

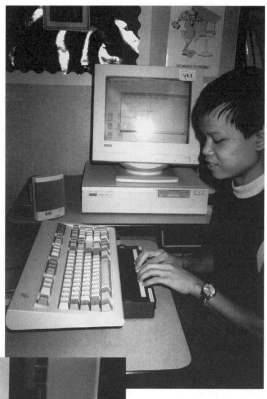

A refreshable braille output that reads line by line from the monitor attached to a PC.

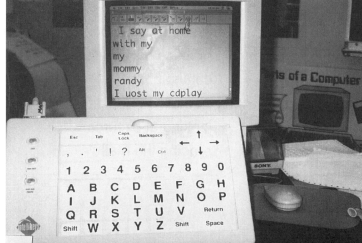

IntelliKeys® with an alphabetical overlay. IntelliKeys® overlays are provided with the device, but any number of overlays can be created for individual and specific purposes. This makes the IntelliKeys® one of the most widely used communication devices and alternative keyboards.

Enlarging Systems and Devices

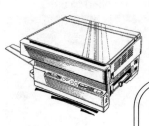

Enlarging systems and devices are a method used to provide magnification of print material and allow the student to function as independently as possible.

Types of Enlarging Devices

magnifiers (e.g., handheld, table-top, Compu-Lenz, CCTV)

monoculars

copier with enlarging capabilities

computer software

Sample Activities

read print material/ worksheets

read computer screen

read maps

read and copy boardwork

practice handwriting/ coloring

cutting nails

threading needles

looking at pictures

reading the mail

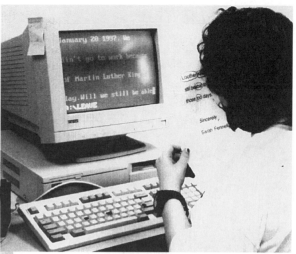

Doing homework with a display that has been adjusted for linespacing and size of print.

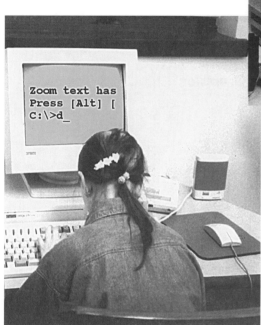

Using Zoomtext® on a PC

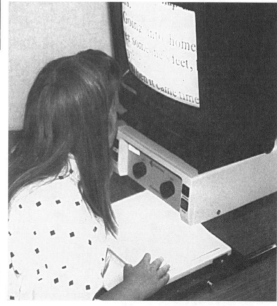

Almost any printed matter can be enlarged on a CCTV.

Tactual Graphics

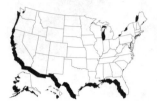

Tactual graphics are raised line or grooved drawings and will have to be created by the paraprofessional or the vision teacher. They reinforce concepts taught in math, science, social studies, and prebraille.

Tools to Create Tactual Graphics*

NOMAD

Picture Braille

Thermoform machine

Stereocopier

Sewell Raised Line Drawing Kit

Tactual Graphics Kit (APH)

Sample Activities

teach tactual
  discrimination skills

teach concepts of page
  orientation

teach map skills

teach graph skills

interpretation of pictorial
  representations

*This list of devices is subject to change depending upon technological advances.

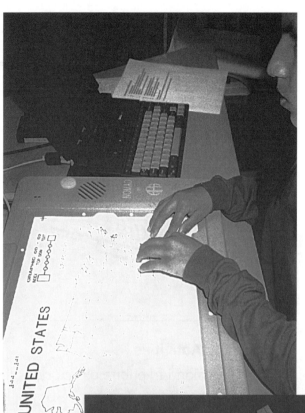

The Nomad® can be programmed specific to the overlay. Here a student learns about the US map.

Graphic adaptations - Clockwise from top left: Bold line graph and writing paper (can be generated on a computer); some tools from the Tactual Graphics Kit (symbols, line wheel, hole punch—which is needed when thermoformed copies are to be made); a representation of a cell using different textures and colors from a biology kit (when the concept is introduced); computer-generated graphics for the Stereocopier (for reinforcement of concepts—braille bar graph and animal tracks); a compass using a serrated wheel instead of a pen (can be used on foil or paper); a template for creating large textured ares (from the Tactual Graphics Kit); a sample of a template to practice one's signature (done on heavy foil which can be reproduced on the Thermoform machine, this template has a grooved and raised outline of the student's name for practice).

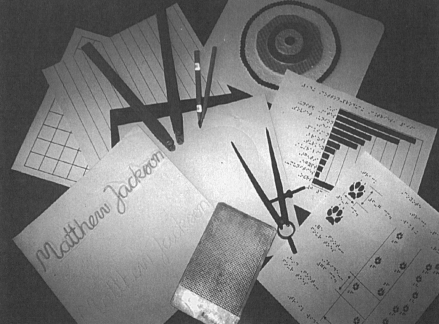

Notetaking Devices

Notetaking devices range from low-tech to high-tech and are used instead of paper and pencil.

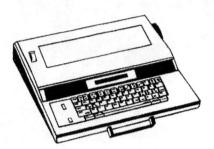

Notetaking Devices*

Slate and stylus
Braillewriter[1]
Braille 'n Speak[1]
Braille Mate[1]
Braille Lite[1]
Braille Desk[1]
BraillePAD[1]
Ergobraille[1]
Type 'n Speak[2]
TransType[2]
SQWERT[2]
MYNA[2]
Keynote[2]
Keynote Companion[2]
MountBatten Brailler[1]
Braille 'n Print[1]/MPrint[1](braille to print devices)
tape recorder

[1]Use braille keyboards
[2]Use regular keyboards

Sample Activities

create calendar, phone directory, lists

take class notes

outline a research report

complete classwork/tests

produce hard copies when needed

some can be used as speech synthesizers (e.g., Braille 'n Speak)

self-management and organization for increased independence

*This list of devices is subject to change depending upon technological advances.

Technology

The Type 'n Speak gives voice output of any type of text.

Laptop computers are available in a variety of styles and can be adapted with speech software.

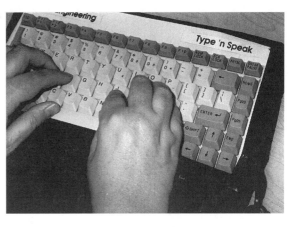

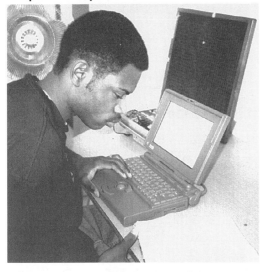

The teacher dictates homework assignments to her student using a Braille Lite.

The slate and stylus needs no batteries and is easy to carry. Special slates for brailling smaller paper and playing cards are also available.

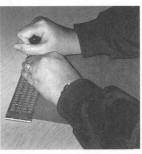

Students who have the use of only one hand may find it easier to use a one-handed brailler that has extended keys.

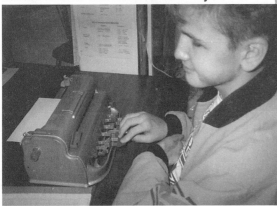

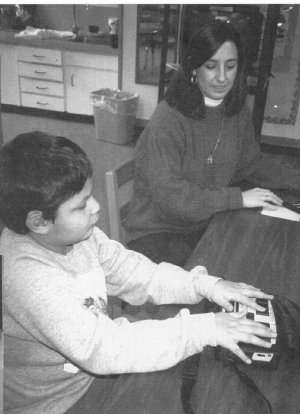

Reference
Systems

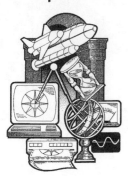

Reference systems allow students to access reference material, such as an encyclopedia, dictionary, and thesaurus.

Types of Reference Systems

electronic talking dictionary

encyclopedia on CD-ROM

on-line library systems

Sample Activities

improve spelling and
language skills

participate in research
activities

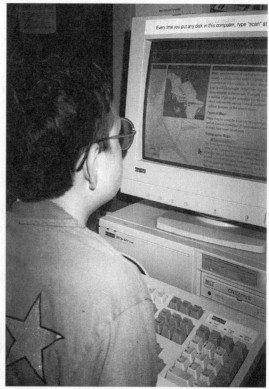

Encyclopedias published on CD-ROM have made it relatively easy for students with low or no vision to access a wealth of information through large print and voice output.

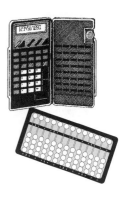

Students can perform math calculations with

- a talking calculator
- a built-in calculator in personal computer
- an abacus

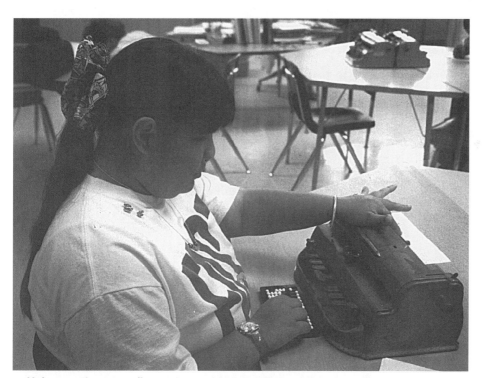

Using an abacus to figure the problem and then writing the answer on the brailler is a low-tech, practical approach to math.

Technology

Computer Systems

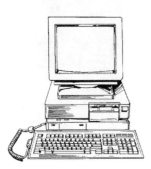

Special computer systems may be necessary to accommodate a student's visual needs or to provide access to the computer screen through speech. Such systems usually include the use of large print and/or speech software. Large print software enlarges text and graphics on the screen. Speech software, also known as screen review software, is used for students whose vision does not allow them to access information on the computer screen through regular or large print. Speech software is also utilized by students who read print but may require speech for back-up. There is also specific software that will allow students to access the Internet.

Examples of Systems and Software*

Large print word processors
Apple	Bank Street Writer
	Kidsword
IBM	Eye Relief
	KV Word
	Big WordPerfect

Screen enlargement software
Apple	Closeview
Macintosh	Closeview
	inLARGE
IBM	ZoomText
	ZoomText for Windows
	MAGic
	MAGic Deluxe
	MAGNUM
	LP-DOS
	LP-DOS for Windows

*This list of devices is a sampling and subject to change depending upon technological advances. It is not intended to be a complete listing of all products currently available.

Technology

Talking word processors

Apple	Dr. Peet's Talk Writer
	BEX
	ProWords
	AppleWorks with AppleWorks companion
	KeyTalk
Macintosh	Write:OutLoud (also has large print capabilities)
	IntelliTalk (also has large print capabilities)
	Kid Works
IBM	Keysoft
	IntelliTalk for DOS

Screen review software (speech software)

Macintosh	outSPOKEN
IBM	ASAP
	ASAW
	Business Vision
	WinVision
	JAWS
	JAWS for Windows
	Vocal Eyes
	Window Eyes
	outSPOKEN for Windows
	Master Touch

Speech synthesizers (in order for screen review software and word processors to *talk*, speech synthesizers are needed; they can be external— attached to the computer—or internal—inside the computer)

Apple	Echo Speech Synthesizer
IBM	Artic SynPhonix
	Artic Transport
	Accent PC and SA
	Sounding Board
	Double Talk
	DECtalk
	Keynote GOLD
	Braille 'n Speak
	Braille Lite
	BraillePAD
	Braille Desk
	TransType
Macintosh	speech is built in

Braille translators (when students need material translated into braille, these programs change print text to braille)

Apple	BEX
Macintosh	Duxbury
IBM	Ransley Interface
	MegaDots
	Duxbury

Braille printers (to print out translated material)

	Braille Blazer
	Braillo
	Thiel
	VersaPoint
	MountBatten
	Romeo
	Juliet

Additional Reading

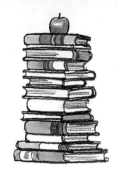

Closing the gap. Published bimonthly. Contact Closing the Gap, PO Box 68, Henderson, MN 56044, Tel. 612-248-3294.

Compton, C. (1989). *Assistive devices: Doorways to independence.* Washington, DC: Assistive Devices Center. Department of Audiology and Speech-Language Pathology, School of Communication, Gallaudet University.

Computer resources for people with disabilities: A guide to exploring today's assistive technology. (1994). Alameda, CA: Hunter House Inc.

Lewis, R. (1993). *Special education technology: Classroom applications.* Pacific Grove, CA: Brooks/Cole Publishing.

Livingston, R. (1997). *Use of the Cranmer abacus.* Austin: Texas School for the Blind and Visually Impaired.

McNairn, P., & Shioleno, C. (1993). *Quick tech activities for literacy.* Wauconda, IL: Don Johnston, Inc.

Rocklage, L. A., Peschong, L. A., Gillett, A. L., & Delohery, B. J. (1996). *Good junk + creativity = great low-end technology.* Ypsilanti, MI: Four Weird Women, Inc.

Technology

Technology

Adaptation

by Chrissy Cowan

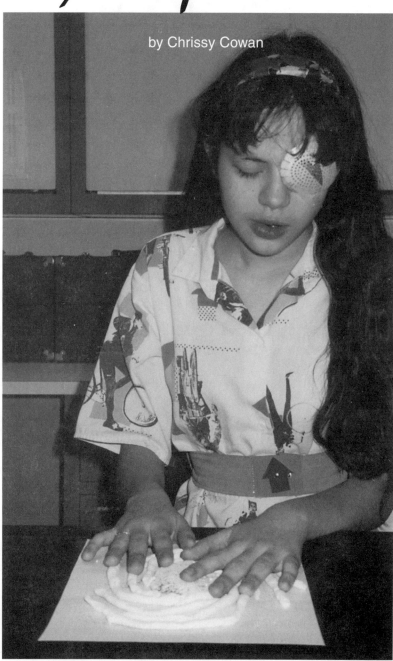

The student is exploring a creative adaptation of a spiral galaxy. This tactual graphic uses styrofoam strips to give the impression of the visual picture seen through high-powered telescopes.

What Materials Needs Adaptation?

Materials and concepts being taught will change according to the age of a student and the curriculum chosen by the school. Lighting needs and visual contrast should be taken into consideration when adapting any materials. The following are examples of places and materials typically used by students which may require modification (e.g., labelled in braille, large print). Refer to the appendix for ordering information on adapted equipment.

Preschool Programs

● Classroom, restroom, and cabinet doors and shelves

● Prereading activities requiring matching, tracking, sequencing

● Learning stations and displays

● Toys and representations of objects

● Early books

- Classroom, restroom, and cabinet doors and shelves

- Pre-braille and braille reading readiness materials

- Learning stations and displays

- Representations of objects

- Early books

- Manipulatives for math

Kindergarten

- Pleasure reading books

- Books and worksheets

- Maps, charts, graphs

- Tapes

- Representations of objects

- Devices used to measure

- Information presented on films, video, computer, TV, overhead projector screens, display charts, and chalkboards

Grades 1-5

Adaptation

Grades 6-12

- Books and worksheets in all subject areas
- Maps, charts, graphs
- Tapes
- Representations of objects
- Devices used to measure
- Information presented on films, video, computer, TV, overhead projector screens, display charts, and chalkboards
- Reference materials
- Fiction and nonfiction reading materials

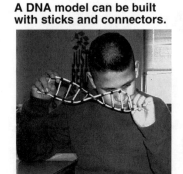

A DNA model can be built with sticks and connectors.

Reading and writing tools - Clockwise from top left: Brailler, magnetic place holders, writing board with string lines and bead markers for indenting, screen board that leaves tactual lines when writing on paper overlays with a crayon or primary pencil, cursive letter template, signature guide, slate and stylus on a clipboard, large braille cell for beads or finger tips, movable pegs to create words, swing braille cell with removable pegs to simulate braillewriter keys and written cell

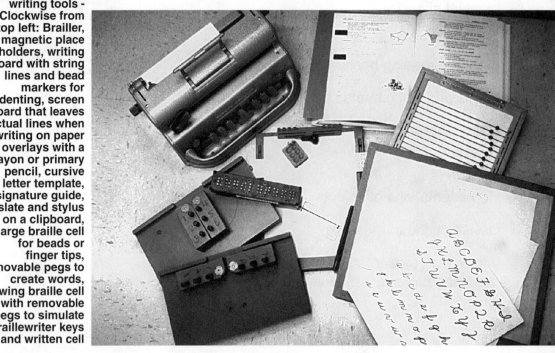

Adaptation

Most textbooks are already available in braille and large print through the American Printing House for the Blind (APH). Braille comes in several codes. Books and other literature are prepared in Grade Two literary braille, which is a combination of individual letters of the alphabet and contracted letters frequently used, such as *ed, sh, th,* etc. In addition, words and parts of words which are frequently used are contracted in the literary braille code. Examples of contracted words are *with, the, and,* and *but.* This code applies a set of rules for when these contractions can be used. Computer software designed to prepare literary braille automatically applies the rules for using the contractions. Another commonly used braille code is called Nemeth code, which is used in the preparation of math books and materials.

Unfortunately, in Texas the mass production of braille and large print ends with state adopted text books and some supplementary materials. Any other material the general education teacher uses to supplement the text, and in some cases, supplant the text, must be prepared by the VI program. Students with low vision who have difficulties with regular print or contrast can enlarge print using magnification devices such as hand-held magnifiers or closed circuit TV sets (CCTV). Teachers can also modify print assignments by enlarging them on a copy machine. Depending on the assignment and individual learning styles, students who are totally blind will require braille, raised tactual drawings (lines, symbols, etc. that can be felt), or audio-taped materials.

Adaptation

Why Is Adaptation Important?

Imagine you are a blind student sitting in your fifth grade classroom as your teacher discusses your next assignment. You will be responsible for researching at least three resources from the library on some aspect of the weather, writing a three-page report, and building a model to present to the class. The adults in your life surely want you to experience success, and they feel it is important for you to be as self-sufficient as you can be. With these goals in mind, they encourage you to express your needs and work with them to complete this assignment.

The vision teacher may have discussed the assignment in advance with the general education teacher and instructed you in the methods for ordering your own research materials on tape. She may have demonstrated the weather concepts as you were learning them in science by acquiring models or tools to help make more abstract concepts such as condensation, clouds, and temperature measurement more concrete so that you could understand them better. In addition, she has been working with you on using the technology needed for just such a project: a variable speed tape recorder, specialized tapes, and an electronic device for brailling your notes, draft, and final report. Worksheets with complicated maps, charts, and graphs would have been provided in a tactual format for you to read. At home your mother and father dig through the garage to find stuff in an effort to help you construct your model of clouds to complete your assignment. In the end, you have not only learned more about your subject, you have also learned to use techniques and tools that will continue to serve you throughout your life. Add to this the benefit of working on an assignment that parallels that of your sighted peers and you emerge as a self-confident and respected classmate.

Within this scenario many adaptations were made that enabled the blind student to benefit from the assignment made by the general education teacher. Some of these adaptations were of materials: special tapes, brailled materials, models, tactual graphics; and some were methods: ordering over the phone, communicating with others, utilizing technology, and writing a rough draft and final report. Typically the vision teacher will be responsible for coordinating this type of learning experience with parents, teachers, the student, and paraprofessionals. Each person plays a role in making learning more meaningful, and allows students with visual impairments to process the same information as their sighted peers.

Adaptation

Due to the inclusion of students with visual impairments into public school settings, the need to adapt curriculum and learning material originally designed for sighted students has become a critical part of the overall programming. Because certified vision teachers work with students ranging in age from infancy through twenty-two, the scope of materials used in individual settings is phenomenal. Vision teachers will also be responsible for programming in areas outside the school setting, such as daily living skills, vocational skills, and recreational skills, which bring with them unique concepts and materials that must be made available and meaningful to students with visual impairments. In addition to the range of ages, grade levels, settings, and curricular areas, the variety of cognitive abilities and degree of visual loss must be considered. Altogether these factors require knowledge of diverse methods for adapting materials.

Braillists create work texts, testing material, and otherwise unavailable printed matter for one or more students.

The Paraprofessional's Role

Vision teachers are skilled at analyzing a given educational task in order to determine the *intent* of the lesson. For example, if a general education teacher wants to teach the beginning sound that the letter *d* makes by giving the students a sheet with pictures of objects to be circled if they begin with the *da* sound, a vision teacher will know that the skill of recognizing the *da* sound is what's important. She may adapt the lesson to include objects, some of which begin with the *da* sound, or a worksheet that has been changed from the original print version. Experience in working with a variety of curricula and age ranges augments the vision teacher's knowledge of how best to adapt material for the subject being studied, and it is not uncommon for the vision teacher, the general education teacher, and paraprofessional to brainstorm together for adaptations to be made for the benefit of the student.

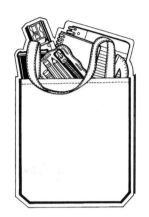

Different ages of students require different formats. Typically a younger child will require simpler formats, or worksheets where information on the page is uncluttered. Often assignments are shortened due to the reduced reading speeds of the students who are blind or have a decreased acuity. The paraprofessional will work closely with general education teachers under the direction of the vision teacher to adapt material. In addition to developing a knowledge base about adapting material, the parapro-fessional will benefit from the ability to communicate with a variety of professionals and students, organize vast amounts of material, and use equipment developed for modifying print into braille and/or a raised line drawing.

Adaptation

Communication

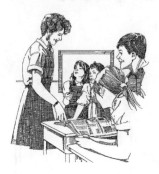

In most situations the vision teacher is itinerant, traveling from school to school or town to town with a typical case load ranging from 10 to 18 students. The paraprofessional will probably either be stationed on the campus where the most blind students are located or in a centrally located office. If you are on the same campus with the blind student(s), it will be most natural for the general education teachers to come to you for suggestions for modifications because you are readily accessible. Hopefully the vision teacher has established a working relationship in which she has communicated the need for material to be adapted in advance of the assigned date for distribution to the students, but there will always be frantic last minute requests from individuals. Handling these requests will require skill and tact, as it will be important not to react in a way that negatively affects the relationship between the general education teacher and the student. Setting up a system to manage requests for material adaptations in advance with all parties involved, including the student, is the most effective method to foster positive communication between professionals.

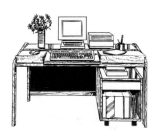

If ever there was an occupation in which the skill of organization is critical, this is the one! There are countless timelines to contend with in addition to the paperwork that will cross your work station. General education teachers should be encouraged to provide material to be adapted at least one week in advance. However, material which includes maps, charts, and graphs is more labor intensive and will require a longer amount of time to adapt. You will be responsible for:

- Organizing a system for receiving and distributing classroom material in a timely fashion

- Storing both current and past projects, keeping an inventory of material on hand

- Keeping track of software and equipment used to make adaptations.

Students with visual impairments and the professionals with whom they work require space for their equipment, books, and papers. The ability to find useful discarded furniture, shelving, and file cabinets also comes in handy.

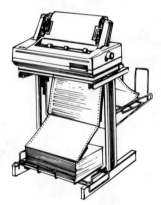

Equipment for Preparing Brailled Material

In order to create the highest quality instructional material, the vision teacher will provide guidelines on the appropriate format and presentation for specific students. With the introduction of software which translates printed input into braille, it is no longer necessary to be able to read braille in order to prepare brailled material. The keyboard used is the standard QWERTY display for typing information to be translated by the software. As with any software there are commands to learn in order to format information being entered. Examples of print-to-braille translation software are MegaDots (for MS-DOS), Duxbury (for Windows and Macintosh) and BEX (for Apple computers). Once the information is keyed in, commands are given to translate into braille and output onto a braille printer. At this time, this is only available for literary translation. However, software for the Nemeth math code translation* is nearing completion.

* by Raised Dot Computing™

Another way to produce braille is on the Perkins Brailler, which is a standard manual braille writer. Its use requires proficiency in both reading and writing in the braille code and formatting rules. The disadvantage of the Perkins is fairly obvious—you have to know the code. However, the advantage is that it allows you the flexibility of creating maps, charts, and graphs (without trying to figure out a computer!), and preparing math papers in Nemeth Code.

The American Printing House for the Blind (APH) markets a prebraille program (*Patterns*) which includes instructions for making tactual readiness books for prereaders. APH also has a *Handbook for Learning to Read Braille by Sight* for learning the basics of braille reading, and *Learning the Nemeth Braille Code: A Manual for Teachers and Students*. Another resource is *Just Enough to Know Better* (National Braille Press).

Adaptation

Equipment for Producing Tactual Drawings and Other Tactual Material

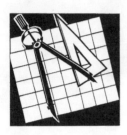

In addition to changing printed material into braille, you will be responsible for changing maps, charts, graphs, and diagrams into a tactual format. A good place to look for ideas and equipment is the APH (American Printing House for the Blind) catalog. The vision teacher should have one available. The equipment used for making tactual conversions can be as simple as a tracing wheel, like the kind used in sewing, or as sophisticated as an electronic device that changes a hand drawn image into one that has raised lines.

- In situations where multiple copies of one graphic is needed, a Thermoform machine is used. This machine uses heat to literally mold a thin sheet of plastic over a sheet of paper bearing braille, raised line drawings, or thin objects (e.g., dried spaghetti).

- Another method is the stereocopier. There is one on the market called Tactual Image Enhancer which enables you to make a raised line drawing by copying your image onto a special type of paper.

- For creating your own raised line graphics, a Tactile Graphics Kit can be ordered at no charge to the school district through quota funds from the American Printing House for the Blind. It contains specialized tools for creating textured surfaces, raised lines, and raised symbols for making maps and graphs.

Adaptation

- For times when a quick and simple modification will do, APH also has a Tactual Graphics Starter Kit which contains material such as craft ink and fabrics and patterns.

- The American Thermoform Corporation markets a product called Braillabel, an adhesive-backed sheet which can be loaded into a Perkins Brailler to make sturdy labels for cassette tapes, CD jackets, cabinet doors, games, maps, canned and boxed food products, crayons, etc. They also market other tactual material.

- A braille labeler is available that does not require knowledge of the braille code, but is limited in the contractions it can produce.

- Game boards and simple maps can be made using cookie sheets or other metal sheets (such as a counter-top protector sold at hardware stores) and magnetic strips or 8 X 10 magnetic sheets which can be cut into shapes. Adapted game pieces can be made by gluing magnets to the bottoms of game pieces so that they are not knocked over as the student with a visual impairment searches for his piece.

Many math adaptations are simple hands-on materials that all students in a math class will appreciate.

- Homemade adaptations are often very effective. Fabric, textured paper, foam-backed plastic placemats, yarn and glue can be used creatively.

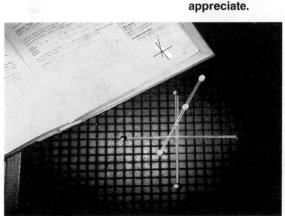

APH Handicassette and APH Variable Speed Recorder

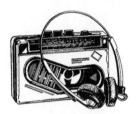

These tape recorders, available on quota funds from the American Printing House for the Blind, are specially designed to play tapes distributed by the Library of Congress Talking Book Division and Recordings for the Blind and Dyslexic. These tapes are recorded on four tracks at half speed and require specialized tape players. The modified players allow the listener to speed up the tapes in a way that does not distort the speech. Both cassette players have the same functions, but the Handicassette is portable and favored by students who change classrooms. Not all visually impaired students can use taped material successfully, and caution should be exercised by the educational team when considering converting print material into an auditory mode. Most students will need instruction in how to use these specialized tape recorders, and the tapes as well.

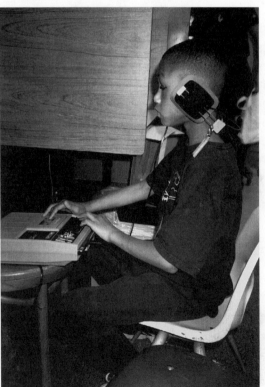

Cassette recorders are available from the American Printing House for the Blind. They give students access to recorded learning material, listening skills practices, and reading for pleasure.

Adaptation

120

Suggestions

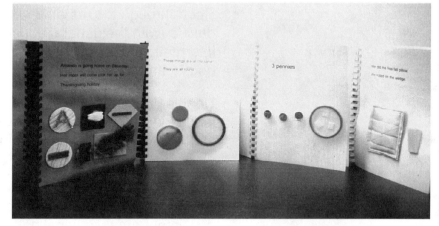

Because the population of students with visual impairments is so small and varied, it may take years of experience to develop an expertise in learning styles and formats that are best for different age groups and abilities. Printed matter developed for young students is made to be colorful, with a variety of formats which include print, pictures, and different arrangements on the page. Unfortunately, the very things that make assignments interesting to a student with sight make them confusing to one without. You, the vision teacher, and the general education teacher will go through a period of trial and error as you explore formats that work best for a particular visually impaired student.

Books that teach basic concepts can be created from readily available material (e.g., for shapes, numbers, textures, simple stories).

A household scale can be adapted by labeling the markings in braille.

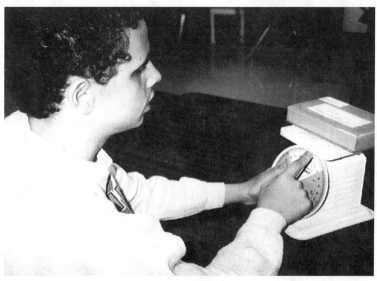

Adaptation

When deciding how to modify a print assignment, the following guidelines may help you with the process:

- Read through the material to be modified and decide (with the general education teacher) which information is absolutely necessary and which can be discarded.

- Double space material for braille readers in grades K-2, older students with lower reading levels, and students of any age just learning braille.

- Avoid clutter, especially on maps and math sheets.

- Avoid random formats. Instead use some sort of consistent organizational pattern such as rows, columns, or numbered problems/sentences.

- All pages should be clearly labeled and numbered if there is more than one so that the blind student can keep papers organized.

- Proofread your work.

- Avoid using all capitals. It is easier for students to read print in upper and lower case.

- Nonserif and nonitalicized fonts are generally easier to read (e.g., Helvetica, Geneva).

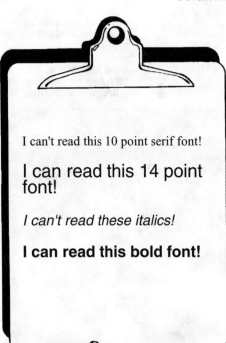

I can't read this 10 point serif font!

I can read this 14 point font!

I can't read these italics!

I can read this bold font!

Adaptation

When preparing tactual graphics, the following guidelines published by the American Printing House for the Blind are helpful:

- Graphics should be tactually clear and contain only relevant information.

- Graphics should be two-dimensional with the possible exception of some mathematical diagrams.

- Avoid clutter and simplify.

- Split complicated graphics into sections or layers of information, with one providing an overview. Replace three-dimensional figures with cross sections or front, top, and side views whenever possible.

- Identify all important features shown on a graphic.

- Place labels in such a manner as to leave the reader in no doubt as to what is being identified.

- Label liberally for orientation (e.g., capitals, bodies of water, etc.).

- Be consistent in using symbols within graphics of the same type.

- Explain and define all symbols, either on same page or facing page.

- Use different tactual symbols for different types of information.

- Separate symbols by at least 1/8 inch.

Adaptation

- Apply the 1/8 inch separation rule to features that are separate, even if doing so introduces some spatial distortion.

- Use two-letter US postal codes where applicable (and other two-letter codes where postal codes are not applicable) for labels on maps.

- Omit capital letters in labels when meaning will not be distorted.

- Use grade two braille contractions in labels.

- A two-cell braille symbol is preferable to a one-cell symbol for labels.

- Do not break the integrity of a shape with a braille label (e.g., the border of a state with its braille label).

- Match map symbols and labels with legend symbols and labels.

- The symbols in the legend should feel like the symbols on the map or other drawing and should not be surrounded by boxes.

- On the map itself, use a directional indicator only where north is not the far edge (i.e., top of page). When north is not the far edge, indicate directionality by using a simple arrow labeled *N*. Avoid using the compass rose. North can also be indicated by a line at the top of the page (e.g., a row of braille c's).

- Position scale and other indicators as consistently as possible, preferably at the top of tactual graphics. When it is necessary to distort the scale, this fact should be indicated in a transcriber's note.

- Place all titles, keys, and legends before the graphic. If there is not room on the page with the graphic, place on opposing page.

Most paraprofessionals learn *on the job* as new challenges present themselves. If you are interested in learning the braille code there are classes available through an extension course, distance education, or sometimes locally. For the truly determined there is a braille transcriber's certificate correspondence course available through the National Library Service for the Blind and Physically Handicapped. See page 155 of the Appendix for the address.

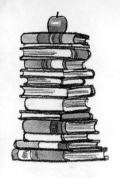

Additional Reading

Olson, M. R. (1984). *Guidelines and games for teaching efficient braille reading.* New York: American Foundation for the Blind.

Torres, I., & Corn, A. C. (1990). *When you have a visually handicapped child in your classroom: Suggestions for teachers.* New York: American Foundation for the Blind.

American Printing House for the Blind Catalog. PO Box 6085, Louisville, KY 40206-0085. Tel. 800-223-1839

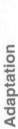

Adaptation

Students With Multiple Impairments

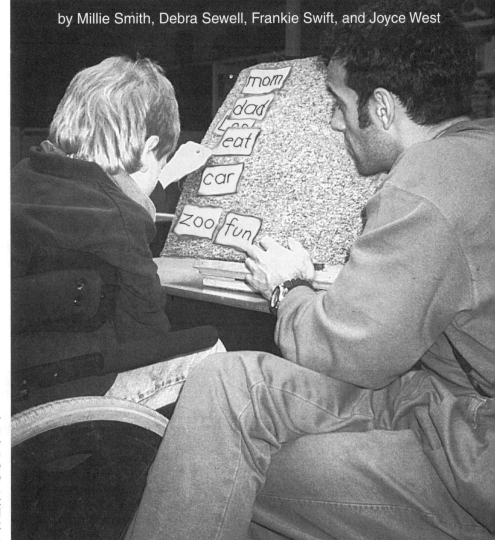

by Millie Smith, Debra Sewell, Frankie Swift, and Joyce West

The para-professional often works on a one-on-one basis with a student who has multiple impairments. Here the student points to word cards to talk about his family.

Who Are Students with Multiple Impairments?

Students with multiple impairments have a range of abilities and skill levels. If the additional impairment(s) affects cognitive functioning, the students' abilities can vary from mild to severe or profound retardation. Thus, some of these students may master functional academics and basic skills while others will learn to maintain alert states more efficiently. Some will have motor and visual impairments only, or speech-language disorders along with vision problems, and have normal cognitive development. There are many kinds of impairments that may be present in addition to a visual impairment. Often, the visual condition reflects one aspect of a genetic syndrome, such as Down's Syndrome, which has multiple effects on the child's functioning. Students who have experienced visual problems as a result of traumatic brain injury, for example, may have other neurological deficits as well. The term multiple impairments itself will not define the level of functioning or the appropriate programming. In this chapter, the discussion will focus on those students with visual and multiple impairments that include cognitive delays.

What Are Important Goals for These Students?

One important goal of instruction is to maximize each student's participation in activities. Students should be encouraged to be independent, although complete independence may not be possible or desired. Too much help may make students unnecessarily dependent.

Students at any cognitive level need to initiate:

- Interactions with adults and peers

- Requests for desired activities

- Functional use of objects for play and work

- Activities related to daily living

- Movement from place to place

If adults anticipate every need, initiate every activity, and sustain all actions within activities, little or no learning can take place.

The Paraprofessional's Role

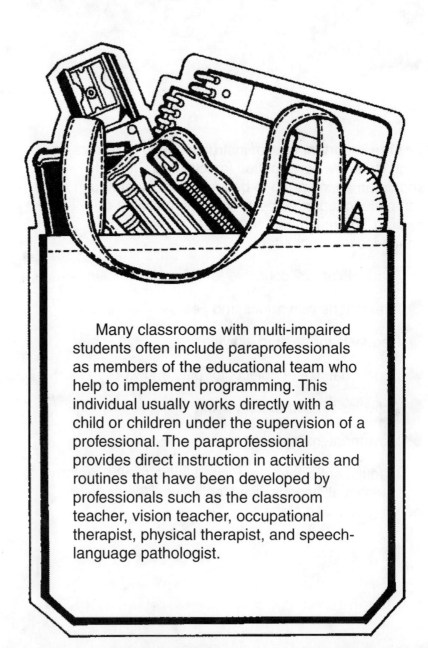

Many classrooms with multi-impaired students often include paraprofessionals as members of the educational team who help to implement programming. This individual usually works directly with a child or children under the supervision of a professional. The paraprofessional provides direct instruction in activities and routines that have been developed by professionals such as the classroom teacher, vision teacher, occupational therapist, physical therapist, and speech-language pathologist.

The paraprofessional implements the instructional strategies of the team by:

- Instructing individual students

- Assisting the teacher in observing, recording, and charting behavior and progress

- Implementing behavior management strategies

- Implementing instructional plans for self-help skills (e.g., buttoning, zipping)

- Implementing instructional plans for recreation/leisure skills

- Implementing instructional plans for vocational skills

- Assisting the teacher with crisis problems and discipline

- Assisting with the preparation of materials

- Assisting students with personal and hygienic care

- Setting up and maintaining special classroom equipment

- Positioning students

- Helping students with assistive devices (e.g., braces, wheelchairs, low vision devices)

- Helping students who need assistance with eating

- Helping students get on and off the bus

- Helping with the development of activities and routines by providing feedback to the team.

Mutliple Impairments

The paraprofessional fosters independence in students by:

- Providing only as much help as is necessary

- Waiting for the students to do the part that they can do

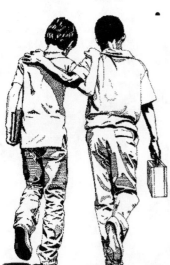

- Helping the students focus on the classroom teacher instead of providing separate instruction

  Reducing adult support by letting peers who are participating in the same activity help whenever possible rather than adults.

The paraprofessional enhances the dignity of the students by:

- Modeling respect

- Asking the students' permission before positioning or handling

- Allowing the students to make choices

- Telling students what is going to happen.

Suggestions

Teaming

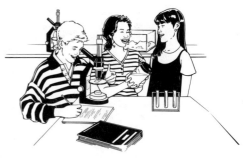

Students with multiple impairments usually have a variety of needs. Therefore, educational programs require a team effort for assessment and instruction. Teams might consist of any of the following members: classroom teacher, parent, vision teacher, orientation and mobility specialist, occupational or physical therapist, speech-language pathologist, certified teacher of auditory impairments, paraprofessional(s), counselor, and nurse.

Sometimes direct instruction needs to be limited to a few members of the team because students have difficulty adjusting to different instructional styles.

Paraprofessionals are significant team members since they spend a large part of the day directly involved with the student. As such, paraprofessionals may be aware of activities that do not appear to contribute to the educational goals or the student's well being. This will need to be reported to the team so that the activity can be modified.

Role Release

Role release is a technique used to help team members share information with each other so that instruction is consistent among many team members. It also allows adaptations and strategies to be integrated into activities occurring throughout the day.
For example:

- The occupational therapist shows the teachers, paraprofessional, parent and speech-language pathologist a procedure for prompting head lift. That procedure is then used throughout the day, across all settings, even when the OT is not present.

- The speech-language pathologist shows all team members how to model appropriate language. That strategy is implemented in all instructional activities and by all adults interacting with the student.

In order to be released to do a specific procedure, the following steps must be followed:

1. The specialist shares information with the team members.

2. The specialist models or teaches the procedure.

3. Each team member gets guided practice in the use of the procedure.

4. Each team member implements the procedures as prescribed.

5. The specialist periodically observes the team members carrying out the activity to make sure that use of the procedure is correct and consistent, and makes changes as needed based on student development.

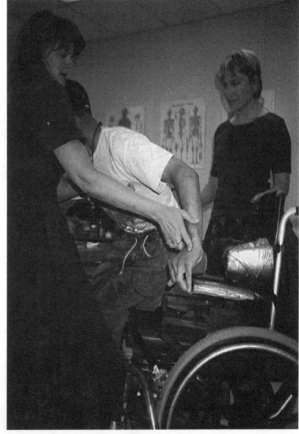

The physical therapist demonstrates a wheelchair transfer to a paraprofessional. She shows how to cue the student when it is safe to let go by lightly touching his hand.

Assessment

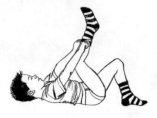

For this population, assessment is best when based on observation of student performance in a variety of activities over time.

1. The whole team, including the parents, must be involved to get a complete picture of how students are functioning.

2. A variety of activities should be observed.

3. Observations must take place over an extended period of time.

4. Multiple locations should be included (e.g., home, classroom, cafeteria, bus) as many students do not generalize skills from one setting to another.

Paraprofessionals may be the only team members directly involved in some activities and may see a greater variety of activities. This observation data is valuable and should be shared. Information may be shared with other team members in the form of informal checklists or daily logs.

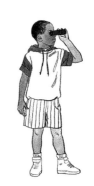

Children who are eligible to receive VI services display a wide range of visual abilities. This range can extend from total blindness to normal vision within a restricted field. Even students with very low vision may respond to some visual stimuli.

Visual abilities may fluctuate for a variety of reasons such as medication levels, seizure activity, and energy levels. Paraprofessionals need to alert the vision teacher or nurse if they observe the following:

- Unusual redness or puffiness in or around the eyes

- Rubbing or scratching around the eyes

- Tearing

- Matting (unusual discharge)

- Complaints of headaches

- Excessive crying or personality changes

- Head banging.

Special Visual Needs

Problems	Suggestions
Is visually inattentive.	Let the student move to stimulate the visual system.
Turns head to side to view objects.	Let the student view object in the best visual field.
Sees something one day/ moment and not able to see it the next.	Believe the student. Use nonvisual alternatives and try a visual approach at a different time.
Does not respond immediately to objects, events.	WAIT! Some students may need from several seconds to a minute or two to process and respond.
Does not respond to stationary objects.	Move objects in preferred viewing area/areas.
Sees objects in one or several different areas (fields) (e.g., tunnel vision, scotomas).	Allow student to tilt/move head or move object. Consult vision teacher about best visual field.
Sees objects better in bright light *or* dim light.	Consult the vision teacher about lighting needs.
Has difficulty seeing a single object in a cluttered space.	Eliminate clutter.
Does not see objects when they blend with background colors.	Increase contrast between the color of object and the background.

Optical Devices

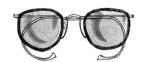

When students have optical devices such as glasses, a magnifier, or a telescope, the paraprofessional needs to actively seek instruction in the appropriate use of these devices from the vision teacher or the O&M specialist.

Paraprofessionals are often involved in helping maximize the benefit of optical devices by doing the following:

- Encourage wearing prescription glasses and using optical devices.

- Clean lenses.

- Report broken optical devices.

- Remove glasses during nap time, sidelying, etc.

- Teach responsible behavior in the care of optical devices to the student.

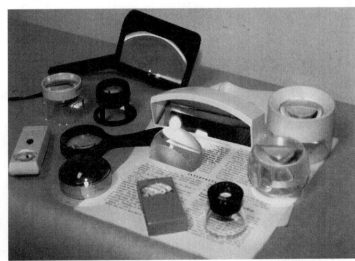

Magnifiers come in all shapes and sizes. Paraprofessionals often play a significant role in ensuring proper care and use of optical devices.

Mutliple Impairments

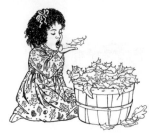

Use of Touch

Many students with visual and multiple impairments learn about their world primarily through touch. They need help learning to:

• Explore and manipulate objects.

• Use tactual symbols for communication.

• Read braille in functional contexts.

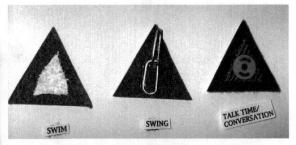

SWIM   SWING   TALK TIME/CONVERSATION

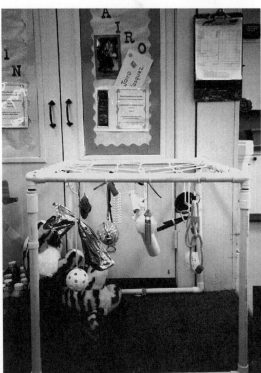

Top: Three tactual symbols for activities from the Standard Tactual Symbol System: a piece of terry cloth for swimming; a chain link for swing; an abstract symbol for talk time.
Center: One version of a "little room" for a small child to explore objects safely.
Bottom: Shown here are a hierarchy of symbols for eating: a spoon (metal or plastic), part of a spoon, the word "eat" in enlarged braille, and in large letters for a student with vision.

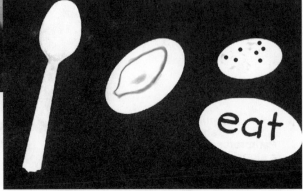

Special Tactual Needs

Problems	Suggestions
Shows little interest in objects.	Make sure that objects have interesting sensory qualities (e.g., textures, sound, bright colors, moving parts, vibration).
Does not use objects appropriately.	Teach and practice appropriate use of objects in meaningful activities.
Resists being touched (tactual defensiveness).	Let the students know they are about to be touched. Introduce material gradually. Stop when students indicate the desire to stop. Use a firm rather than a light touch. Let the students touch you rather than you touching them. If you have to touch the students, do so where they tolerate touch best. Place students at the beginning or end of a waiting line to minimize touching.
Avoids touching objects.	Do not force students to touch objects when they are resistant. Provide objects that have tactual qualities pleasing to students (e.g., hard surfaces, vibration, heaviness). Avoid manipulating students' hands as much as possible.

Here tactual symbols are used in a daily calendar book: a silk flower for Earth Works (a horticultural unit), a bell for music, a string circle for circle time. The days of the week each have their own distinct symbol: Tuesday - tic-tac-toe, Wednesday - bottle cap, Thursday - pipe cleaner, Friday - sponge.

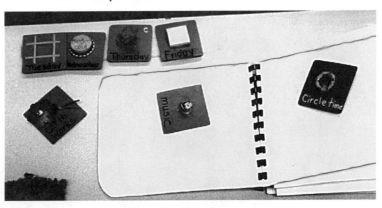

Movement

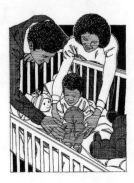

Students with visual and multiple impairments may have delayed motor development because:

- Motivation to move is reduced because they don't see objects and events in their environments.

- Sometimes well-intentioned adults help too much by bringing objects to them rather than expecting them to find and move to objects.

- They may be afraid to move out into space.

Encouraging Movement

- Provide opportunities for vestibular experiences (e.g., treadmill, merry-go-round, rocking chair).

- Make sure the student moves to an object. Do not bring the object to the student if at all possible.

- Define safe, familiar play and work spaces.

- Provide a stimulating environment so that the student has a reason to move.

- Make sure objects are consistently left in the same place so the student can learn where they are and actively retrieve and replace them.

Mutliple Impairments

Positioning for Optimal Sensory Experiences

Students with multiple impairments often need physical support to maintain the head and trunk control necessary to access their environment. This is an important component of the program, as correct positioning is critical to help the student use the vision, hearing, and tactual senses effectively. Ongoing consultation from occupational and physical therapists and the vision teacher on the team is necessary to ensure appropriate positioning throughout the day.

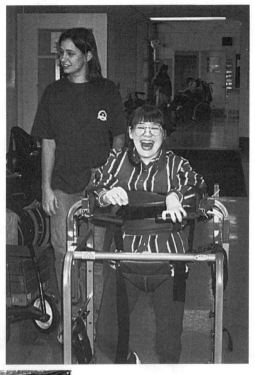

This student enjoys spending time out of her wheelchair. The paraprofessional accompanies her while letting her explore the school's hallways and other general areas.

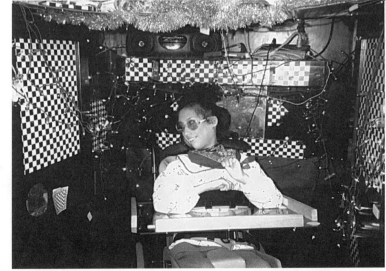

This version of a "little room" was designed for older students who operate switches to turn on lights and sounds. The patterns and colors are used to stimulate vision; sound can be used to calm the student. By letting the student operate the lights and sounds, she can control her environment.

Mutliple Impairments

143

Communication

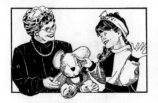

All children communicate. Paraprofessionals can help students learn communication skills by making sure they have many opportunities to communicate. For example, before providing a drink, ask the student if he wants a drink and wait for a response. Another way to increase communication is to provide choices.

Communication skills tend to encourage appropriate behavior so children don't have to rely on primitive communication methods like tantrums, crying, or aggression. Many students with visual and multiple impairments use these alternative forms of communication:

• Object symbols

• Signs/gestures

• Picture boards

• Tactual symbols

• Voice production devices

Some students may have difficulty using some of these alternatives. Following are adaptations that have worked with students who have visual and multiple impairments. It is important to work with the educational team to identify appropriate adaptations for effective communication.

Examples of Problems and Suggestions for Adaptations

- If the student does not understand or cannot see pictures, substitute objects where pictures are usually used.

- If the student has limited ability to see details, modify pictures by highlighting the most important parts or use objects and tactual symbols instead of pictures.

- If the student cannot see picture symbols, use tactual symbol cards made by gluing objects or parts of objects on a card.

- If the student cannot see signs and gestures because of too much figure-ground clutter, wear a solid color vest or wear gloves to highlight hands when signing to the student. Modify signs if they are presented outside the student's field of vision. Use tactual signs if the student has no vision.

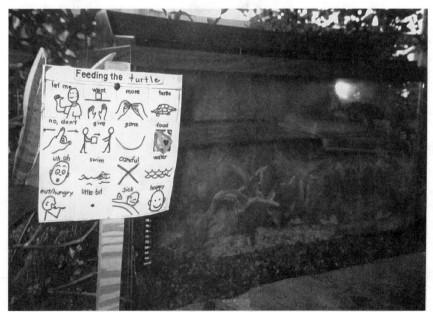

A picture board in the hall can prompt students to communicate. Feeding a turtle, for example, can be a positive reinforcement when on the way to an activity the student does not like to do.

145

Echolalia

Some students may have a problem known as echolalia. Echolalic students may repeat words, phrases and sentences and sometimes whole stories without understanding the meaning of the words they use. It is important to work with the vision teacher and speech-language pathologist to ensure appropriate programming for students who are echolalic. However, these general guidelines might be helpful:

- Reduce verbal input. Talk less, not more.

- Use language directly related to concrete experiences (e.g., don't tell a student what a dog is without having a real dog present).

- Let the student generate comments. Expand on the comments rather than initiating all the language yourself.

- Help reinforce the use of communication by responding to the meaning even when the student has not used the correct words.

Calendars

Students with visual and multiple impairments who have little or no vision may need object-based communication systems. One system for this is an object calendar. Students use a display to represent time; usually this starts with a series of boxes. Objects are placed in the boxes to represent activities. In this way, students without vision learn to use objects to anticipate and talk about the activities of the day. Some students use pictures or tactual symbols in calendars as their communication skills become more symbolic. Calendar systems should be set up and carried out under the supervision of a vision teacher and/or speech-language pathologist who has had training in this method.

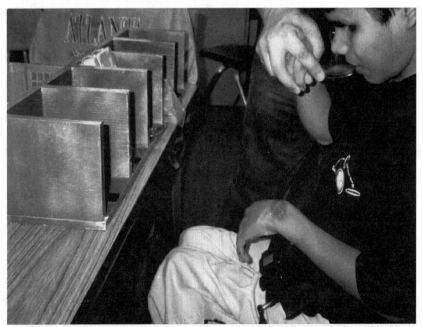

This student is using the calendar box with a *finished box* placed behind it (to prompt to reach). Object symbols are a spoon for eating (metal spoons are sturdier and should belong only to a particular student), a toothbrush for brushing teeth, a book for schoolwork, a plastic bag for toileting, and a ball for playtime.

Environmental Adaptations

Students with visual and multiple impairments need structure and consistency in their environments:

Problems	Suggestions
Lack of consistency in the environment	Keep objects, furniture, etc. in designated areas.
Large wide open spaces	Give landmarks to help them orient themselves in space.
Clutter	Reduce or limit the number of objects in work areas.
Lack of room organization	Organize work areas with only the objects needed for a specified task.
Disorganized tasks	Set up tasks the same way (e.g., left to right).
Lack of attention to objects	Light the object; use high contrast, bright colors to draw attention to objects.
Glare	Watch out for laminated material, shiny surfaces, light coming through windows, and direction of artificial lighting.
Doors left partially open	Remember to keep doors open all the way or closed so students won't run into them when trailing a wall.
Different kinds of lighting is needed for different visual conditions	Ask the vision teacher to determine the unique lighting needs for your students.

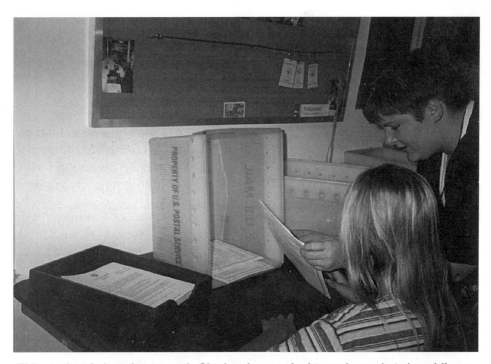

This student is learning to work. She has been asked to make packets by adding a cover letter to a stapled stack. The job coach is showing her the sequence: Take the letter from the tray; next comes the stapled stack; place the combined stack at the right. Assemblies with clear sequences are often used to introduce students to the world of work. The bulletin board above this workstation has an added feature, *finished* symbols strung on a line. In this case the symbols represent each day she works during one week.

Behavior

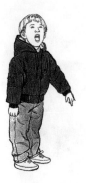

Many students will have a behavior management plan developed by the team that you will help to implement. Here are some common behaviors related to vision loss that may be interpreted as noncompliance:

Common Behaviors	Possible Reasons
Throws objects.	Tactual defensiveness (see page 141). Reluctance to hold objects. May be using sound cues to get information about the environment beyond reach.
Refuses to move.	Insecure about where they are being asked to move to.
Removes or tears clothing, or hits people when touched.	Tactual defensiveness. Lack of tolerance for being touched.
Appears to ignore instructions.	Students without vision may not know they are being addressed unless their names are used.
Continually talks even when the class is expected to be quiet.	Silence may cause anxiety when students cannot see what is happening.

There are other behaviors, known as stereotypical behaviors, frequently observed in children with visual impairments. These may include rocking, eye poking, flicking, and spinning. These behaviors often result from lack of sufficient and appropriate stimulation.

It is important to redirect stereotypical behaviors. Telling students to "stop" is not effective. Students must be given an alternative that is more acceptable. The team needs to develop a strategy for dealing with these behaviors.

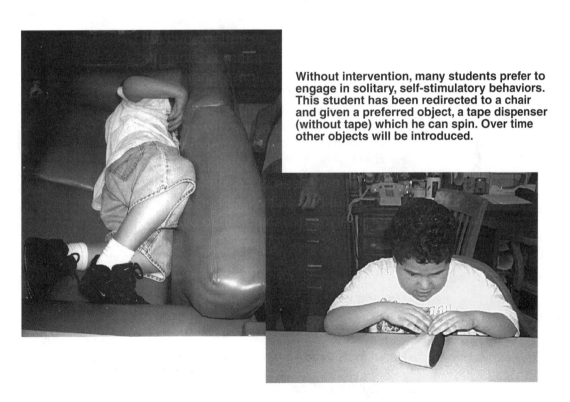

Without intervention, many students prefer to engage in solitary, self-stimulatory behaviors. This student has been redirected to a chair and given a preferred object, a tape dispenser (without tape) which he can spin. Over time other objects will be introduced.

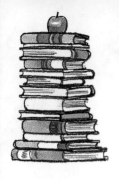

Additional Reading

Brennan, V., Peck, F., & Lolli, D. (1992). *Suggestions for modifying the home and school environment: A handbook for parents and teachers of children with dual sensory impairments.* Watertown, MA: Perkins School for the Blind.

Brody, J., & Webber, L. (n. d.). *Let's eat: Feeding a child with a visual impairment.* Los Angeles: Blind Children's Center.

Chen, D., & Dote-Kwan, J. (1995). *Starting points: Instructional practices for children with multiple impairments including visual impairments.* Los Angeles: Blind Children's Center.

Hug, D., Chernus-Mansfield, N., & Hagaski, D. (n. d.). *Move with me: A parents' guide to movement and development for visually impaired babies.* Los Angeles: Blind Children's Center.

Kekelis, L., & Chernus-Mansfield, N. (1984). *Talk to me II: Common concerns.* Los Angeles: Blind Children's Center.

Kekelis, L., & Chernus-Mansfield, N. (1984). *Talk to me: A language guide for parents of blind children.* Los Angeles: Blind Children's Center.

Meyers, L., & Lansky, P. (n. d.). *Dancing cheek to cheek: Nurturing beginning social, play and language interactions.* Los Angeles: Blind Children's Center.

Recchia, S. (n. d.) *Learning to play: Common concerns for the visually impaired preschool child.* Los Angeles: Blind Children's Center.

Appendix

Addresses for Ordering Adapted Material and Equipment

American Foundation for the Blind, 11 Penn Plaza, Suite 300, New York, NY 10001, Tel. 212-502-7661: products for low vision and tactual consumers and professional publications.

American Printing House for the Blind, Inc., PO Box 6085, Louisville, KY 40206-0085, Tel. 800-223-1839: Teaching material and equipment.

American Thermoform Corporation, 2311 Traverse Avenue, City of Commerce, CA 90040, Tel. 800-331-3676: Equipment and supplies for braille reproduction.

Ann Morris Enterprises, Inc., 890 Fams Court, East Meadow, NY 11554-5101, Tel. 800-454-3175: Innovative products for people with vision loss.

Carolyn's Products for Enhanced Living, 5603 Manatee Avenue W., Bradenton, FL 34209, Tel. 800-648-2266: Equipment and supplies for daily living.

Howe Press, Perkins School for the Blind, 175 North Beacon Street, Watertown, MA 02172: Instructional aids.

Independent Living Aids, Inc., 27 East Mall, Plainview, NY 11803-4404, Tel. 800-537-2118: Can-Do Products; aids and appliances for personal and professional uses.

The Lighthouse Inc., 36-20 Northern Boulevard, Long Island City, NY 11101, Tel. 800-829-0500: Products to help people with impaired vision.

LS & S Group, Inc., PO Box 673, Northbrook, IL 60065, Tel. 800-468-4789 or 847-498-9777: Personal and professional products for persons with a visual and/or hearing impairment.

Maxi-Aids, 86-30 102nd St. Richmond Hill, NY 11418, Tel. 800-522-6294 or 718-846-4799: Low vision and other optical devices, daily living appliances and tools.

National Library Service for the Blind and Physically Handicapped, Braille Development Section, 1291 Taylor Street NW, Washington, DC 20542, Tel. 800-424-8567: Information regarding Braille Transcriber's Certification.

Repro-Tronics, Inc., 75 Carver Ave., Westwood, NJ 07675: Tactile Image Enhancement Products, *Bumpy Gazette* (newsletter).

Texas State Library, Division for the Blind and Physically Handicapped, Capitol Station, PO Box 12927, Austin, TX 78711, Tel. 800-252-9605: Regional library providing talking books, braille, and large type books, cassette books. *Note: Library of Congress affiliated state or regional libraries may be contacted for these services.*

Printed Resources

The materials in this list were selected because they provide a theoretical basis for the importance of focusing on specific areas or because they offer practical suggestions for implementation. All of the publications are specific to programming for students who are visually impaired.

Overview

Bishop, V. E. (1996). *Teaching visually impaired children.* 2nd ed. Springfield, IL: Charles C. Thomas.

Hagood, L. (1997). *Communication: A resource guide for teachers of students with visual and multiple impairments.* Austin: Texas School for the Blind and Visually Impaired.

Levack, N. (1994). *Low Vision: A resource guide with adaptations for students with visual impairments.* 2nd ed., Austin: Texas School for the Blind and Visually Impaired.

Scholl, G. T. (Ed.). (1986). *Foundations of education for blind and visually handicapped children and youth: Theory and practice.* New York: American Foundation for the Blind.

Smith, M., & Levack, N. (1996). *Teaching students with visual and multiple impairments: A resource guide.* Austin: Texas School for the Blind and Visually Impaired.

Social Skills

Bishop, V. E. (1986). Identifying the components of successful mainstreaming. *Journal of Visual Impairment & Blindness, 80,* 939-946.

Chen, D., Friedman, C. T., & Calvello, G. (1989). Learning together: A parent guide to socially-based routines for visually impaired infants. In *Parents and visually impaired infants.* Louisville, KY: American Printing House for the Blind.

Cushman, C. (1992). Social development. In C. Cushman, K. Heydt, S. Edwards, M. J. Clark, & M. Allon, *Perkins activity and resource guide: A handbook for teachers and parents of students with visual and multiple disabilities* (v. 1). Watertown, MA: Perkins School for the Blind.

Davidson, I. F., & McKay, D. K. (1980). Using group procedures to develop social negotiation skills in blind young adults. *Journal of Visual Impairment & Blindness, 74*, 3, 251-255.

Davidson, I. F., & Simmons, J. N. (1984). Mediating the environment for young blind children: A conceptualization. *Journal of Visual Impairment & Blindness, 78* , 6, 251-255.

Fazzi, D. L., Kirk, S. A., Pearce, R. S., Pogrund, R. L., & Wolfe, S. (1986). Social focus: Developing socioemotional, play, and self-help skills in young blind and visually impaired children. In R. L. Pogrund, D. L. Fazzi, & J. S. Lampert (Eds.), *Early focus: Working with young blind and visually impaired children and their families* (pp. 50-69). New York: American Foundation for the Blind.

Harrell, R. I., & Strauss, F. A. (1986). Approaches to increasing assertive behavior and communication skills in blind and visually impaired persons. *Journal of Visual Impairment & Blindness, 80*, 6, 794-798.

Hazekamp, J., & Huebner, K. M. (Eds.). (1989). Unique educational needs related to a visual impairment. In *Program planning and evaluation for blind and visually impaired students: National guidelines for educational excellence* (pp. 8-14). New York: American Foundation for the Blind.

Hoben, M., & Lindstrom, V. (1980). Evidence of isolation in the mainstream. *Journal of Visual Impairment & Blindness, 74*, 289-292.

Huebner, K. M. (1986). Social skills. In G. T. Scholl (Ed.), *Foundations of education for blind and visually handicapped children and youth* (pp. 341-362). New York: American Foundation for the Blind.

Loumiet, R., & Levack, N. (1993).*Independent living: A curriculum with adaptations for students with visual impairments. Vol. I: Social competence.* Austin: Texas School for the Blind and Visually Impaired.

MacCuspie, P. A. (1996). *Promoting acceptance of children with disabilities: From tolerance to inclusion.* Halifax, Nova Scotia: Atlantic Provinces Special Education Authority.

Mangold, S. S. (1982). Nurturing high self-esteem in visually handicapped children. In *A teacher's guide to the special needs of blind and visually handicapped children.* New York: American Foundation for the Blind.

Mangold, S. S. (1988). Nurturing high self-esteem in adolescents with visual handicaps. *Journal of Vision Rehabilitation, 2,* 3, 5-9.

McCallum, B. J., & Sacks, S. (Eds.) (n. d.). *Santa Clara County social skills curriculum for children with visual impairments.* B. J. McCallum, 1296 Mariposa Ave. San Jose, CA 95126.

Parsons, S. (1987). Locus of control and adaptive behavior in visually impaired children. *Journal of Visual Impairment & Blindness, 77,* 6, 261-268.

Read, L. F. (1989). An examination of the social skills of blind kindergarten children. *Education of the Visually Handicapped, 20,* 4, 142-155.

Sacks, S., Gaylord-Ross, R., & Kekelis, L. (1992). *The development of social skills by blind and visually impaired students.* New York: American Foundation for the Blind.

Simmons, J. N., & Davidson, I. F. (1984). Mediating the environment for young blind children: An introduction to the literature. *Journal of Visual Impairment & Blindness, 78 ,* 3, 118-120.

Swallow, R. M., & Huebner, K. M. (Eds.). (1987). *How to thrive, not just survive.* New York: American Foundation for the Blind.

Tuttle, D. W., & Tuttle, N. R. (1996). *Self-esteem and adjusting with blindness: The process of responding to life's demands.* Springfield, IL. Charles C. Thomas.

Appendix

Van Hasselt, V. B., Hersey, M. S., Kazdin, A. E., Simon, J., & Mastanuono, A. (1983). Training blind adolescents in social skills. *Journal of Visual Impairment & Blindness, 77*, 5, 199,203.

Daily Living Skills

Broom, S., Leader, P., Maher, B., & McCallum, B. J. (n. d.). *Santa Clara County personal management for independent living.* Santa Clara, CA: SCORE Regionalization Project. B. J. McCallum, 1296 Mariposa Ave., San Jose, CA 95126.

Condon, R. (1992). *Toilet training children with deaf/ blindness/multiple disabilities: Issues and strategies.* Unpublished handout. Outreach Department Texas School for the Blind and Visually Impaired, 1100 West 45th St., Austin, TX 78756.

Crawford, J. L. (1993). *Techniques and adaptations for teaching eating skills with the blind.* Kansas City: Kansas State School for the Blind.

Crawford, J. L. (n. d.). *Techniques and adaptations for teaching housekeeping skills with the blind.* Kansas City: Kansas State School for the Blind.

Dickman, I. R. (1986). *Making life more livable: Simple adaptations for the homes of blind and visually impaired older people.* New York: American Foundation for the Blind.

Edwards, S. N. (1992). Independent living skills. In. C. Cushman, K. Heydt, S. Edwards, M. J. Clark, & M. Allon, *Perkins activity and resource guide: A handbook for teachers and parents of students with visual and multiple disabilities.* Vol. 1. Watertown, MA: Perkins School for the Blind.

Ferrell, K. A. (1985). *Reach out and teach: meeting training needs of parents of visually and multiply handicapped young children.* New York: American Foundation for the Blind.

Loumiet, R., & Levack, N. (1993). *Independent living: A curriculum with adaptations for students with visual impairments*. 2nd ed. Vol. II. Austin: Texas School for the Blind and Visually Impaired.

Mangold, P. N. (1980). *The pleasures of eating for those who are visually impaired*. Castro Valley, CA: Exceptional Teaching Aids.

Swallow, R. M., & Huebner, K. M. (Eds.). (1987). *How to thrive, not just survive: A guide for developing independent living skills for blind and visually impaired children and youths*. New York: American Foundation for the Blind.

Woodward, C. (n. d.). *Sewing techniques to use with visually handicapped or totally blind students*. Unpublished manuscript. Available from TSBVI Curriculum, 1100 West 45th St., Austin, TX 78756.

Yeadon, A. (1974). *Toward independence: The use of instructional objectives in teaching daily living skills to the blind*. New York: American Foundation for the Blind.

Orientation and Mobility Skills

Dodsun-Burk, B., & Hill, E. W. (1989). *An orientation and mobility primer for families and young children*. New York: American Foundation for the Blind.

Eigler, J. (n. d.). *Preschool learning and mobility: How parents can help in training the very young blind child in orientation and mobility*. Unpublished manuscript.

Hill, E. W., & Ponder, P. (1976). *Orientation and mobility techniques: A guide for the practitioner*. New York: American Foundation for the Blind.

Huebner, K. M., Prickett, J. G., Welch, T. R., & Joffee, E. (Eds.). (1995). *Hand in hand: Essentials of communication and orientation and mobility for students who are deaf-blind*. 2 vol. New York: American Foundation for the Blind.

Appendix

Jacobson, W. (Ed.). (1993). *The art and science of teaching orientation and mobility to persons with visual impairments.* New York: American Foundation for the Blind.

Lydon, W. T., & McGraw, M. L. (1973). *Concept development for visually handicapped children.* New York: American Foundation for the Blind.

O'Mara, B. (1989). *Pathways to independence.* New York: The Lighthouse, National Center for Vision and Child Development.

Pogrund, R., Healy, G., Jones, K., Levack, N., Martin-Curry, S., Martinez, C., Marz, J., Roberson-Smith, B., & Vrba, A. (1993). *TAPS: An orientation and mobility curriculum for students with visual impairments.* Austin: Texas School for the Blind and Visually Impaired.

Smith, A. (1992). *Beyond arm's reach: Enhancing distance vision.* Philadelphia: Pennsylvania College of Optometry Press.

Swallow, R. M., & Huebner, K. M. (Eds.). (1987). *How to thrive, not just survive: A guide for developing independent living skills for blind and visually impaired children and youths.* New York: American Foundation for the Blind.

Students With Multiple Impairments

Alsop, L. (Ed.). (1993). *A resource manual for understanding and interacting with infants, toddlers, and preschool age children with deaf-blindness.* Logan: SKI•HI Institute, Department of Communicative Disorders, Utah State University.

Brennan, V., Peck, F., & Lolli, D. (1992). *Suggestions for modifying the home and school environment: A handbook for parents and teachers of children with dual sensory impairments.* Watertown, MA: Perkins School for the Blind.

Chen, D., & Haney, M. (1995). An early intervention model for infants who are deaf-blind. *Journal of Visual Impairment & Blindness, 89,* 5, 213-221.

Chen, D., Friedman, C. T., & Calvello, G. (1989). *Parents and visually impaired infants (PAVII).* Louisville, KY: American Printing House for the Blind.

Cushman, C., Heydt, K., Edwards, S., Clark, M. J., & Allon, M. (1992). *Perkins activity and resource guide: A handbook for teachers and parents of students with visual and multiple disabilities.* 2 vol. Watertown, MA: Perkins School for the Blind.

Efron, M., & DuBoff, B. R. (1976). *A vision guide for teachers of deaf-blind children.* Raleigh: North Carolina Department of Public Instruction.

Erin, J. (1990). *A unique learner: A manual for instruction of the child with visual and multiple disabilities.* Austin, TX: Education Service Center, Region XIII.

Goetz, L., Guess, D., & Stremel-Campbell, K. (Eds.). (1987). *Innovative program design for individuals with dual sensory impairments.* Baltimore: Paul Brookes.

Hagood, L. (1997). *Communication: A resource guide for teachers of students with visual and multiple impairments.* Austin: Texas School for the Blind and Visually Impaired.

Harrell, L., & Akeson, N. (1987). *Preschool vision stimulation: It's more than a flashlight.* New York: American Foundation for the Blind.

Harring, N. G., & Romber, L. T. (Eds.). (1995). *Welcoming students who are deaf-blind into typical classrooms: Facilitating school participation, learning, and friendship.* Baltimore: Paul H. Brookes.

Huebner, K. M., Prickett, J. G., Welch, T. R., & Joffee, E. (Eds.). (1995). *Hand in hand: Essentials of communication and orientation and mobility for your students who are deaf-blind.* 2 vol. New York: American Foundation for the Blind.

Appendix

Korsten, J. E., Dunn, D. K., Foss, T. V., & Francke, M. K. (1994). *Every move counts.* San Antonio, TX: Therapy Skills Builders.

Langley, M. B. (in press). *Individualized, systematic assessment of visual efficiency for the developmentally young individual (SAVE).* Louisville, KY: American Printing House for the Blind.

Levack, N., Hauser, S., Newton, L., & Stephenson, P. (1996). *Basic skills for community living: A curriculum for students with visual and multiple impairments.* Austin: Texas School for the Blind and Visually Impaired.

Morgan, E. C. (1992). *The INSITE model: Resources for family-centered intervention for infants, toddlers, and preschoolers who are visually handicapped.* 2 vol. Logan: SKI•HI Institute, Department of Communicative Disorders, Utah State University.

Nielsen, L. (1993). *Early learning, step by step in vision impaired and multiply handicapped children.* Copenhagen, Denmark: SIKON.

Rowland, C., & Schweigert, P. (1990). *Tangible symbol systems: Symbolic communication for individuals with multisensory impairments.* Tucson: Communication Skill Builders.

Smith, A. J., & Cote, K. S. (1984). *Look at me: A resource manual for the development of residual vision in multiply impaired children.* Philadelphia: Pennsylvania College of Optometry Press.

Smith, M., & Levack, N. (1996). *Teaching students with visual and multiple impairments. A resource guide.* Austin: Texas School for the Blind and Visually Impaired.

Snell, M. E. (Ed.) (1993). *Systematic instruction of the moderately and severely handicapped.* 4th ed. Columbus, OH: Charles Merrill.

Appendix

Ain't Misbehavin'

This video discusses strategies for interpreting and dealing with challenging behaviors of students who are deafblind. Texas School for the Blind and Visually Impaired, Outreach Dept., 1100 West 45th St., Austin, TX 78756-3494.

Bringing Out the Best: Encouraging Expressive Communication and Getting in Touch

These two videos focus on interrupted routines, touch and object cues, and other communication strategies with children with multiple disabilities including those who are deafblind. Research Press, 2612 N. Mattis Ave., Champaign, IL 61821.

Can Do! Video Series

Video 1 Seeing Things in a New Way: What Happens When You Have a Blind Baby.

Video 2 Learning About the World: Concept Development.

Video 3 Becoming a Can-Do Kid: Self-Help Skills.

Video 4 Making Friends: Social Skills and Play.

Video 5 Going Places: Orientation and Mobility.

This series is designed to teach parents in a friendly and non-intimidating way. Six families of visually impaired children, ranging in age from 14 months to six years old, model in their own homes some basic and important practices in parenting a visually impaired child. Several blind adult role models provide inspiration for the future as they discuss their experiences and feelings about growing up blind. Visually Impaired Preschool Services, Inc., 1215 S. Third Street, Louisville, KY 40203.

Functional Vision: Learning to Look

This video uses real life examples to explain how parents can help children with visual impairments develop skills for searching, finding, following, shifting attention and integrating eye-hand movements. BVD Promo Services, P.O. Box 931082, Verona, WI 53593-0182.

Getting in Touch

This videotape is designed to introduce parents and others working with sensory impaired children to some basic principles to help make communication go more smoothly. Research Press, 2612 N. Mattis Ave., Champaign, IL 61801.

Getting There: A Look at Early Mobility Skills of Four Young Blind Children

This video highlights instructional strategies and mobility skills for four young children who are blind. Blind Babies Foundation, 1200 Gough St., San Francisco, CA 94104.

Hand in Hand

A one hour introduction for family members and others on strategies for working with individuals who are deafblind. Can be used alone in whole or part, or with the *Hand in Hand* written resources. American Foundation for the Blind, Eleven Penn Plaza, Suite 300, New York, NY 10001.

Let's Eat: Feeding a Child with a Visual Impairment

This video presents a variety of techniques to help families teach competent feeding skills to their young children with visual impairments. Blind Children's Center, 4120 Marathon St., Los Angeles, CA 90029.

Making the Most of Early Communication

Presents selected strategies for communicating with infants, toddlers, and preschoolers whose multiple disabilities include vision and hearing loss. Emphasis is placed on ways to improve information through activities that are natural, meaningful and motivating. California State University, Northridge, Dept. of Special Education, 18111 Nordhoff, Northridge, CA 91330-265.

Observing and Enhancing Communication Skills for Individuals with Multi-Sensory Impairments

A manual and two video tapes on observing, analyzing, and developing the communication skills of infants, proeschoolers, school-aged students, and adults who have multiple disabilities. Psychological Corporation Order Service Center, PO Box 839954, San Antonio, TX 78283-3954.

SKI*HI Coactive Sign Systems

Video tape 1 Family: Identifying members of the family; Foods.

Video tape 2 Daily Routines: Eating; dressing, undressing; toileting and diapering.

Video tape 3 Daily Routines: Washing and bathing, brushing teeth and combing hair, getting up and going to bed.

Video tape 4 Daily Routines: Play and sensory stimulation; Feelings: Being sick

Video tape 5 Daily Routines: Action words in daily routines; More action words and prepositions in daily routines.

Video tape 6: Going places and visiting people; Special words for visually impaired people.

Video tape 7: Unit 1 - toys & animals; Unit 2 - body parts; Unit 3 - colors; Unit 4 - letters & numbers; Unit 5 - home; Unit 6 - food; Unit 7 - being sick & getting hurt; Unit 8 - time.

Video tape 8: Unit 9 - prepositions; Unit 10 - clothing; Unit 11 - cooking & eating; Unit 12 - pronouns; Unit 13 holidays; Unit 14 - bedroom bathroom; Unit 15 - family & people; Unit 16 - vehicles, places, & things outside.

Video tape 9: Unit 17 - descriptors, adjectives, adverbs, & articles; Unit 18 - going to school; Unit 19 - to be verbs & helping verbs; Unit 20 -action words.

These videos offer a comprehensive training program for learning how to use coactive signing with children who are deafblind. Hope, Inc. 809 North 800 East, Logan, UT 84321.

Appendix

SKI*HI Signals and Cues Series

Video tape 1: Encouraging child to relate to people; Letting child know who you are and what you will do; Deciding what signals and cues to use; A model for using signals and cues.

Video tape 2: Skill: anticipation, Activity: eating or feeding.

Video tape 3: Skill: awareness of child's signals; Activity: toileting, bathing, and brushing teeth

Video tape 4: Skill: giving your child choices; Activity: playing and action; Skill: using Coactive signs; Activity: placing and calming your child.

Video tape 5: Skill: enriching activities and routines; Activity: expressing feelings and using senses; Skill: encouraging active communication; Activity: going somewhere.

These videos offer a wealth of information and techniques for using signals and cues for communication with children who have visual and multiple impairments. 809 North 800 East, Logan, UT 84321.

Appendix

SKI*HI Using Tactile Interactive Conversational Signing

Video tape 1: Topic 1 - Encouraging independent signing: moving from coactive to interactive signing; Topic 2 - Establishing a foundation for conversational interaction: encouraging the child to sign interactively; Topic 3 - Suggestions to encourage language development : vocabulary.

Video tape 2: Topic 4 - Suggestions to encourage language development: using comments, directions, and questions; Topic 5 - Creating a communicative environment: using calendar systems; Topic 6 - Creating a communicative environment: encouraging independence and providing rich language opportunities.

Video tape 3: Topic 7 - Selecting materials and activities that promote interaction; Topic 8 - Establishing guidelines for effective communication; Topic 9 - Conveying emotions and meaning through tactile signs; Topic 10 - Fingerspelling.

Video tape 4: Topic 11 - Encouraging interaction with peers and others within the community; Topic 12 - Interpreting for the individual who is deafblind.

Video tape 5 Topic 13 - Perspectives from individuals who are deafblind.

These videos offer a comprehensive training program for signing with children who are deafblind. Hope, Inc. 809 North 800 East, Logan, UT 84321.

Tangible Symbol Systems

Video and accompanying manual demonstrate the use of objects to communicate about events, people, and things. Communication Skill Builders, PO Box 42050-Y, Tucson, AZ 85733.

What Can Your Child See

Video explains the kinds of vision tests that can be given to infants and young visually impaired children with multiple disabilities. Also demonstrates many interventions for encouraging visual abilities. California State University, Northridge, Dept. of Special Education. 18111 Nordhoff, Northridge, CA 91330-265.

Index

Appendix

S

safety 45, 53
screen enlargement software 100
screen review software (speech software) 101
seating 68
self-advocacy 37
self-concept 21, 59
self-confidence 111
self-help skills 131
self-sufficient 110
senses 14
sensory experience 61
sensory training 53, 60
sequencing 89
setting guidelines 40
sighted guide 54, 67
sighted peers 26
social interaction 22, 29
social skills 20
special tactual needs 141
special visual needs 138
specific techniques 54, 59
speech synthesizers 102
speech-language pathologist 5, 11
spreading with a knife 41
stereocopier 118
strategies 82
stress 50
success 110
suggestions 15, 24–29, 56, 83, 121, 133
switches 86
symbols 145
systematic teaching 36, 43, 84

T

Tactile Graphics Kit 118
tactual cues 63
tactual defensiveness 61, 150
tactual discrimination 90
tactual drawings 118-119
tactual graphics 94, 123-125
tactual image enhancer 118
tactual material 118
tactual needs 141
tactual systems 9, 140, 141
talking word processors 101
tape recorders 120
teams 2, 35, 54, 81, 113, 130, 133
textbooks 109
Thermoform 118
toddlers 72
toileting and hand washing 38
toothbrushing 38
touch 9, 13, 25, 57, 140
toys 61
trailing 66
training 23
transportation 50
travel skills 50
travel techniques 52, 64
tunnel vision 6
turn-taking 26, 86

U

use of senses 9
use of touch 140
use of vision 7
using pronouns 12

V

verbalism 10
VI services 137
video training material 166-178
vision 9-10, 14
vision impairment 6–14, 52
visual abilities 137
visual cues 22
visual feedback 12
visual field 6
visual needs 138
visual observation 22
visual tasks 7
voice output 88

W

worksheets 111

Appendix

176